# Regulating Medicines in Europe

T0203727

*Regulating Medicines in Europe* explains and investigates how medicines are controlled in Europe, especially the EU. Basing their book on penetrating documentary and interview research with the pharmaceutical industry, regulators and consumer organisations, John Abraham and Graham Lewis provide the first major critical examination of the new Europeanised systems of medicines regulation. They argue that the drive to produce and approve more drugs more quickly for a single European market dominates other considerations, such as improvements in democratic accountability, the independence of regulators and scientific expertise from commercial interests, and drug safety testing and surveillance.

The authors demonstrate that national regulatory agencies now compete in an internal EU market for fees from pharmaceutical companies in the race to approve new drugs. The implications of this competition and European harmonisation of risk-benefit assessments for new drugs safety standards, industry–regulator relations and public accountability are carefully scrutinised.

*Regulating Medicines in Europe* will prove a valuable resource to all those concerned with medicine regulation.

**John Abraham** is Professor of Sociology and Co-director of the Centre for Research in Health and Medicine, University of Sussex. **Dr Graham Lewis** is a writer and consultant on European and international medicines regulation, and former Research Fellow in Science Policy, University of Reading.

# Regulating Medicines in Europe

Competition, expertise and
public health

John Abraham and
Graham Lewis

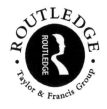

London and New York

First published 2000
by Routledge
2 Park Square, Milton Park, Abingdon, Oxon, OX14 4RN

Simultaneously published in the USA and Canada
by Routledge
711 Third Avenue, New York, NY 10017

*Routledge is an imprint of the Taylor & Francis Group, an informa business*

© 2000 John Abraham and Graham Lewis

Typeset in Sabon by Taylor & Francis Books Ltd

British Library Cataloguing in Publication Data
A catalogue record for this book is available from the British
Library

Library of Congress Cataloging in Publication Data
Abraham, John
Regulating medicines in Europe: competition, expertise, and public
health/John Abraham and Graham Lewis.
p. cm.
Includes bibliographical references and index.
1. Drugs–Testing–Government policy–European Union countries.
2. Drugs–Safety regulations–European Union countries. I. Lewis,
Graham. II. Title.

RM301.27 .A273 2000
353.9'9828'094–dc21                              00-028615

ISBN 978-0–415–20877–2 (hbk)
ISBN 978-0–415–20878–9 (pbk)

# Contents

# Illustrations

## Tables

# Acknowledgements

Our research for this book began in 1994 and was completed in 1999. We are particularly grateful to the UK Economic and Social Research Council (ESRC) who funded much of our research from 1994 to 1997 under its Research Programme in the European Context of UK Science Policy (ESRC Grant No. L323253012). Special thanks go to Peter Healey and the staff at the Science Policy Support Group, who managed and directed that Research Programme. We are also very grateful to all those who participated in our research by giving up their time to be interviewed and/or to provide us with valuable documents and contacts. Many thanks also to Tim Reed, Mike Charlton, Graham Dukes, Heather Gibson, Fiona Bailey, Lauren Dallinger and Michelle Bacca for their support, assistance and co-operation.

# Abbreviations and acronyms

| | |
|---|---|
| ABPI | Association of the British Pharmaceutical Industry |
| ACT UP | AIDS Coalition To Unleash Power |
| ADR | Adverse Drug Reaction |
| ADRC | Adverse Drug Reaction Committee (Sweden) |
| ADROIT | Adverse Drug Reactions On-line Information Tracking Unit |
| AMG | Arzneimittelein Gesetz (German drug law) |
| BEUC | European Consumers' Association |
| BfArM | Bundesinstitut fur Arzneimittel und Medizinprodukte (Federal Institute for Medicinal Products and Devices – current regulatory agency – Germany) |
| BGA | Bundesgesundheitsamt (former German regulatory agency) |
| BIRA | British Institute for Regulatory Affairs |
| BMA | British Medical Association |
| BOD | Board of Drugs (Sweden) |
| BPI | Bundesverband der Pharmazeutischen Industrie e.V. (German industry association) |
| CA | Consumers' Association (UK) |
| CADREAC | Collaboration Agreement of Drug Authorities in European Union Associated Countries |
| CECG | Consumers in the European Community Group |
| CIOMS | Committee for the International Organisation of Medicines (WHO) |
| CMR | Centre for Medicines Research |
| CPMP | Committee for Proprietary Medicinal Products (EEC/EU) |
| CRF | case report form (for individual patients/subjects) |

| | |
|---|---|
| CRM | Committee on the Review of Medicines (UK) |
| CSD | Committee on the Safety of Drugs (UK) |
| CSM | Committee on Safety of Medicines (UK) |
| CTC | Clinical Trial Certificate (UK) |
| DoH | Department of Health (UK) |
| EEA | European Economic Area |
| EEC | European Economic Community |
| EFPIA | European Federation of Pharmaceutical Industry Associations |
| EFTA | European Free Trade Area |
| EMEA | European Agency for the Evaluation of Medicinal Products (EU) |
| EPAR | European Public Assessment Report (EMEA) |
| EPVRG | European Pharmacovigilance Research Group (EU) |
| EU | European Union |
| FDA | Food and Drug Administration (US) |
| FOIA | Freedom of Information Act (US) |
| FOTP | Freedom of The Press Act (Sweden) |
| GAO | Government Accounting Office (US) |
| GATT | General Agreement on Tariffs and Trade |
| HAI | Health Action International |
| ICH | International Conference on Harmonisation of Technical Requirements for Registration of Pharmaceuticals for Human Use |
| IFPIA | International Federation of Pharmaceutical Industry Associations |
| ISDB | International Society of Drug Bulletins |
| JCP | Joint Committee on Prescribing (UK) |
| LIF | Lakesindustrieforeningen (Swedish industry association) |
| MCA | Medicines Control Agency (current regulatory agency – UK) |
| MEDDRA | Medical Dictionary for Regulatory Activities (EU) |
| MINE | Medicines Information Network (EU) |
| MPA | Medical Products Agency (current regulatory agency – Sweden) |
| MRFG | Mutual Recognition Facilitation Group (EU) |
| NAS | new active substance |
| NBHW | National Board of Health and Welfare (Sweden) |
| NCC | National Consumer Council (UK) |

| | |
|---|---|
| NCE | new chemical entity |
| NICE | National Institute for Clinical Excellence (UK) |
| NHS | National Health Service (UK) |
| PCHRG | Public Citizen Health Research Group (US) |
| PL | Product Licence (UK) |
| PMS | Postmarketing Surveillance |
| R and D | Research and Development |
| SBA | Summary Basis of Approval (US FDA) |
| SLA | Department of Drugs (former Swedish regulatory authority) |
| UK | United Kingdom |
| US | United States of America |
| VFA | Verband Forschender Arzneimittelherstellar e.V. (German industry association) |
| WHO | World Health Organisation |
| WTO | World Trade Organisation |

# Introduction

This book is about how medicines are controlled in the European Union (EU), with particular emphasis on the sociology and political economy of medicines regulation. It is written to be accessible to specialists and non-specialists in academia, government agencies, industry, the medical profession and consumer organisations. The focus is on the safety and effectiveness of drug products themselves, rather than on the pricing of medicines. Problems concerning the risks and benefits of medicines are inevitably part of such regulation and involve medical scientists and scientific expertise. Hence, the book may also be seen as an exploration of the relationship between regulation and science. Some may read it as a case study of the pharmaceutical sector in the politics of regulation or European studies, others may read it as a study of regulation within medical sociology, and still others will see it simply as an addition to the literature on medicines policy.

In examining the control of medicines in the EU, we critically discuss the regulatory developments in both individual European countries and EU institutions and systems. Such developments have occurred, and are occurring, against a background of European integration and moves towards a single European market. In that context, harmonisation of medicines regulation within the EU is, of course, a salient issue and is a central part of the Europeanisation of medicines control. While there have been some improvements in the regulation of medicines in Europe, especially in terms of a reduction in wasteful duplication of regulatory work, we argue that it is biased towards the interests of industry and trade over and above the interests of patients and public health. The drive to produce and approve more drugs quickly on to a single European market dominates other considerations such as improvements in democratic accountability, the independence of regulators and scientific expertise from commercial interests, drug safety testing and surveillance, and defining and developing drugs which genuinely meet therapeutic needs, as distinct from those which are marketable.

We are aware that these issues are not confined to the EU. Developments in the EU are frequently influenced by more international or even global considerations. Indeed, institutions of the EU may be pressurised by global institutions to fall into line with international priorities, particularly on matters of trade, even if public health is at stake. For example, in the late 1990s, the World Trade Organisation (WTO) judgement condemning the EU's restrictions on the use of hormones in beef production hinged on the fact that the EU had acted on the basis of consumer fears of health risks in the absence of what the WTO considered adequate scientific testing (Holmes 1999). In the field of pharmaceuticals, however, the EU has taken the lead in the harmonisation of regulatory standards across the world. In other words, on balance, the EU is influencing global medicines regulation more than it is constrained by the regulatory developments in other parts of the world.

Perhaps the most important example of this is in the work of the International Conference on Harmonisation of Technical Requirements for Registration of Pharmaceuticals for Human Use (ICH) during the 1990s. In this context, the North American and Japanese regulators and pharmaceutical industries tend to have followed harmonisation initiatives concerning drug testing standards introduced by their EU counterparts. As a result, the drug regulatory authorities in the US and Japan are obliged to apply the same scientific/regulatory standards when reviewing a wide range of pre-clinical and clinical testing conducted by pharmaceutical companies (see Chapter 5).

Prior to the ICH, the US drug regulatory agency, the Food and Drug Administration (FDA), required that clinical testing for all drugs, whether domestic or imported, should be performed in the US. For example, in the mid-1980s the FDA declared that it regarded foreign clinical data as 'too precarious' for making marketing approval decisions. However, under the ICH, the FDA has agreed to accept some foreign clinical testing. By 1995, the agency had approved some drugs whose clinical trial database was entirely foreign, and established an Office of International Policy and an Office of International Affairs to facilitate international regulatory co-ordination (Vogel 1998). In addition, in 1997 the European Commission reached mutual recognition agreements on standards for good manufacturing practices with Australia, New Zealand, Canada and the US (Anon 1997k), and established mutual recognition agreements on standards for inspections of pharmaceutical industry sites with the US, due to come into operation in 2001 (Anon 1997f).

The primary reason for the EU's influential role in global harmonisation of regulatory standards for medicines is that it is already far advanced in that type of process *because of harmonisation within the EU itself.* Increasingly, European harmonisation goes beyond the EU. In 1998, the drug regulatory authorities of ten Central and Eastern European countries – Bulgaria, the Czech Republic, Estonia, Hungary, Latvia, Lithuania, Poland, Romania, the Slovak Republic and Slovenia – signed up to the Collaboration Agreement of Drug Regulatory Authorities in European Union Associated Countries (CADREAC). Under the latest version of this, these countries have agreed to mutually recognise drug approvals under what is known as the EU's centralised procedure (see Chapter 4).

The implication of these developments in Central and Eastern Europe, North America, Australasia and Japan is that the regulation of medicines in the EU is likely to have ramifications around the globe. Understanding the social science of medicines regulation in the EU may be extremely instructive in assessing regulatory policy developments in other regions of the world. Thus, readers concerned primarily with, say, American drug regulation may also find this book of considerable importance. Furthermore, there are signs that global harmonisation of the pharmaceutical sector may be regarded as a 'test-bed' for other economic sectors.

In Chapter 1, we develop a theoretical framework which guides us in formulating penetrating and meaningful research questions about European medicines regulation. To do this, we draw on concepts from the political economy of regulation, science and technology studies, medical sociology and drug policy studies. The rationale for our empirical research design and the research methods used are discussed in the second chapter. The following five chapters analyse our findings under a set of key issues.

In Chapter 3, we focus on medicines regulation at the 'national level' by investigating the situation in three individual European countries: Germany, Sweden and the UK. After outlining the structure of the key organised interests, such as the pharmaceutical industry and consumer organisations, this chapter traces the development of modern national drug regulation in each European country. Among other things, this demonstrates the nature of the relatively recent convergence of these countries' regulatory regimes towards what we characterise as 'neo-liberal corporate bias'.

The pharmaceutical industry's interest in transnational medicines regulation in Europe (and beyond) is sketched in Chapter 4, where we also introduce and explain the development of the Europeanised systems of medicines regulation, including processes of harmonisation. Chapters 5–7 demonstrate that neo-liberal corporate bias has been reformulated at the 'EU level', albeit in a much more complex form. We then consider the consequences of this for scientific expertise, regulatory science, public health and democratic accountability of medicines regulation. In Chapter 8, we revisit some of the theoretical issues raised in Chapter 1 in order to explain more comprehensively the character of medicines regulation in Europe. Finally, we outline some political implications of our analysis.

# Chapter I

# Science, technology and regulation

In market economies there exists 'a perpetual tension between the freedoms conferred by the private ownership of productive property and the need to impose communal limits on the exercise of those freedoms' (Hancher and Moran 1989a: 1). Regulation is a central way in which governments attempt to manage that tension. In pharmaceuticals, regulatory activity has implications for public health because much of it is concerned with the potential risks and benefits of drugs to patients. Scientific expertise plays a central role in the drug regulatory process.

In this chapter, we discuss several interrelated fields of study pertinent to the examination of medicines regulation: political economy; regulatory science; citizenship; drug development; and public health. Together these provide a theoretical framework which both guides and locates specific research questions. Many of those questions are developed in the concluding section of the chapter.

## Political economy of regulation

The nature of regulation in market economies is highly contested, as indeed is the nature of the state of which government regulatory authorities are part. Few would question that, for analytical purposes, government regulation may be regarded as state intervention in the market, though in reality regulation also creates and circumscribes markets. As such, the 'regulatory state' affects the interests of producers and consumers in the marketplace (Majone 1994). In particular, regulatory activity impacts on private industry. There is also agreement that regulation is generally introduced because of the inadequacies of an unregulated market. However, there the consensus ends. Whether regulation was, is or should be introduced to protect consumer interests over producer interests or vice versa is controversial. Indeed, the definitions of consumer and producer interests, and hence how they are related to the goals of regulatory agencies, are often disputed.

In the US, government regulation of private industry as a response to market failure dates back to the late nineteenth century, with the establishment of a federal agency to regulate the railways. Regulation was seen as a way of promoting efficiency gains. Throughout the twentieth century, many other federal agencies responsible for the regulation of private industries were to follow, including the Food and Drug Administration (FDA) in 1927. By contrast, in Europe until the 1980s the predominant response to market failures was to nationalise private industries (Majone 1996: 9–19). It is not surprising, therefore, to find that the early theories of regulation and regulatory agencies emanate from the US. However, this does not imply that they are irrelevant to analyses of regulation in Europe because, since the 1980s, many countries in Europe have, in some ways, moved towards an American style of regulation. Moreover, despite claims that the market fails to deliver medicines that patients need, few Western European countries have nationalised their *pharmaceutical* industries.

Probably the best-known theory of regulation is that of regulatory capture epitomised by the 'life-cycle' theory of regulatory agencies put forward by Bernstein (1955). According to this theory, regulatory agencies are established as a result of legislation designed to protect certain groups in society against the abuses of industry. It is assumed that there exists some divergence – if not conflict – of interests between industry, seeking to maximise profits, and 'the public interest'. Where 'the public interest' relates to an invisible mass of inactive public, then it is implicitly defined by the objective to correct market failures, such as monopoly power, insufficient information to consumers and inadequate provision of public goods (Majone 1996: 28–9).

Alternatively, 'the public interest' might be defined in relation to the actions of some organised consumer or advocacy group. Typically, legislation will be passed in response to widespread concerns of the wider public, perhaps expressed by consumer interest groups. On this view, therefore, regulatory agencies are set up by the legislature in order to protect the public interest against the excesses of industrial power. Initially, regulatory agencies tend to be aggressive and adversarial towards industry, but become isolated as their enthusiastic staff tire and retire. Eventually they are progressively 'captured' by, and come to share the perspectives of, the industries they are supposed to regulate. From this stage onwards, argues Bernstein, the regulatory agency prioritises industrial interests over consumers, unless or until a scandal highlighting the failures of regulation triggers a new drive for public interest regulation, in which case the regulatory agency begins a new cycle.

Writing from an American perspective, Owen and Braeutigam (1978) provide some interesting insights into how the process of regulatory capture might be operationalised. In a 'how-to' manual for industry, they put forward strategies that they believe might be useful for firms 'playing the regulation game'. Two of these strategies, lobbying agency officials and co-opting expert advisors to regulatory agencies, may be regarded as indicators of capture if they are aimed at diverting agencies' activities away from the protection of the public interest towards the interests of a particular firm or industry. On lobbying regulatory agencies, these authors give the following advice to regulated firms:

> Effective lobbying requires close personal contact between the lobbyists and government officials. Social events are crucial to this strategy. The object is to establish long-term personal relationships transcending any particular issue. Company and industry officials must be 'people' to the agency decision-makers, not just organisational functionaries. A regulatory official contemplating a decision must be led to think of its impact in human terms, and not in institutional or organisational terms. Officials will be much less willing to hurt long-time acquaintances than corporations. Of course, there are also important tactical elements of lobbying, of which not the least is information gathering at low levels of the agency staff. Each contact must be carefully tailored to the background and personality of the official being lobbied. For this reason it is useful to keep files on the backgrounds of agency officials.
>
> (Owen and Braeutigam 1978: 6–7)

Analyses emphasising the importance of trust and experiential judgement over 'knowledge and rational choice' among regulators lend some support to the viability of this advice (McDonell 1997).

Recognising that regulatory policy is effected with the

participation  of experts (often academics), firms are also advised to co-opt these experts, whenever possible, as follows:

> This is most effectively done by identifying the leading experts in each relevant field and hiring them as consultants or advisors, or giving them research grants and the like. This activity requires a modicum of finesse; it must not be too blatant, for the experts themselves must not recognize that they have lost their objectivity and freedom of action. At a minimum, a programme of this kind reduces the threat that the leading experts will be available to testify or write against the interests of the regulated firms.
>
> (Owen and Braeutigam 1978: 7)

How far this advice reflects the attempts by American firms to capture regulatory agencies and the extent to which experts and agency officials succumb to such strategies is an empirical question to which the answer is often unclear. Theoretically, however, such industrial strategies are certainly consistent with the phenomenon of agency capture.

The final indicator of capture, which we shall discuss here, is the 'revolving door' or 'pantouflage' relationship between industry and regulatory agencies (Braithwaite 1986: 298; Hancher and Moran 1989b: 288). This refers to a subculture within leading organisations in the regulatory process in which officials begin their careers as regulators, but then move on to join the industry, or begin their careers in industry, then work for some years in the regulatory agency until they are promoted back into the higher echelons of industry. The 'revolving door' can contribute to capture in at least two ways. If regulators have a background of training in industry, they may be more likely to bring values to the agency which are sympathetic to the regulated industry than if they received training outside industry. More importantly, if regulators see their career development in terms of future promotion into the regulated industry, then they may be unduly concerned to maintain 'friendly relations' with industry at the expense of public interest regulation.

Theories of regulatory capture are often referred to as 'public interest theories of regulation' because they assume that, at the outset, regulation was established in order to serve the public interest, and that its proper role is to continue to do so (Mitnick

1980). Another strand of American political thought, called 'private interest theories of regulation' (also known as 'economic theories of regulation'), takes an altogether more sceptical, if not cynical, view of regulatory agencies and their origins.

For private interest theorists, regulatory agencies do not need to be captured, because they were created to serve the interests of the industries they regulate, especially by helping them to achieve monopolies in the market (Stigler 1971). Far from supporting the public interest against the regulated industry, regulatory measures are enacted and implemented in the interests of specialist producer groups. In exchange for beneficial regulation, private interests must be prepared to deliver votes and resources to political parties. According to Peltzman (1976) politicians and governments wish to maximise vote margins and so use the powers of regulatory agencies to benefit groups that can supply these vote margins. It follows from this that politicians and regulators, who feel less secure in their jobs, are more vulnerable to the influence of private interest groups (Peacock 1984: 17).

Not all groups in society are equally well placed to manipulate the regulatory process. Interest groups, whose members are in good communication with each other, are well-informed and focused on specific demands and command significant material resources, are more likely to be able to influence regulatory agencies than less organised groups. Private interest theorists argue that producer groups that is, private industry – are generally better placed in these respects than consumers. While industry groups may be too small to offer enough votes directly, they can provide valuable resources, including money, which politicians can use to finance their electoral campaigns. However, Peltzman (1976) notes that, if a regulatory agency operates exclusively in the interests of a producer group, then that is likely to arouse opposition from other groups adversely affected by such regulatory policies. Consequently, he proposed that regulatory outcomes are determined by the balance of these opposing interests – the 'political equilibrium' depending on the organisation costs faced by the competing groups. Similarly, Wilson (1980) argues that if the benefits of regulation are diffused but the costs are concentrated on private interests, then regulatory intervention is likely to stall; if the benefits are concentrated on a private interest group but the costs are diffused, then regulation serves the interest group; and if both costs and benefits are concentrated between competing interest groups, the regulator acts as an arbitrator.

Both capture and private interest theories of regulation may be regarded as forms of pluralist theories of the state in the context of European political thought. According to pluralist theory, interest groups compete for resources and success in the political marketplace from which they derive their power to influence government. As Schmitter (1974: 96) explains, pluralism is a system of interest representation in which no interest group exercises a monopoly of representational activity and interest groups are not specially recognised or subsidised by the state. An important corollary to this is that the pluralist state has no independent interests. As interest groups compete for access to government, the state acts as a 'referee' in resolving the demands of the different groups – one-way bargaining from interest group to the state (Cawson 1986: 29–37).

Evidently, pluralist theories of the state conceptualise regulatory agencies as passive and 'black box' them, underplaying the complex institutional environments in which regulators operate (Majone 1996: 30; Mitnick 1980: 111–15). Particularly in the European context, these aspects of pluralist theory have been seen as problematic, leading to a growth in attention to corporatist theories of the state. Unlike pluralism, corporatism implies a 'strong state' which is capable of resisting capture by interest groups. While the corporatist state is not powerful enough to dictate policies to interest groups, bargaining is two-way, involving the state in asserting its own interests. Interest 'intermediation' is also different from pluralism because it involves interest groups, which are non-competitive and which are granted a deliberate representational monopoly by the state in exchange for certain controls on them (Schmitter 1974: 93–4).

According to Cawson (1986: 38),

> corporatism is a specific socio-political process in which organisations representing monopolistic functional interests engage in political exchange with state agencies over public policy outputs which involves those organisations in a role which combines interest representation and policy implementation through delegated self-enforcement.

Such self-regulation is typically achieved by 'social closure' of the kind exhibited by professions or large firms with specialist expertise. Corporatist policy-making may be attractive to the regulatory state because large firms or other interest groups possess 'reservoirs of expertise', whose integration into the implementation of regulation is virtually a precondition for its success (Hancher and Moran 1989b: 272). Moreover, from the perspective of the liberal democratic state, corporatism can help to pacify interest organisations whose economic stakes far outweigh their electoral representation. Typically, such corporatism has been identified with European nation states, such as Sweden and, to a lesser extent, Germany.

The strong regulatory state envisaged by corporatist theories implies that regulatory agencies are not passive, but have their own institutional interests. The characteristics of these interests are undertheorised in the literature, but several possibilities can be readily hypothesised. One option is to revert to public interest theories of regulation by postulating that regulatory agencies have an interest in consumer or public protection derived from the statutes enacted by the legislature that created the agencies. Another is to apply Marxist theories of the state, which imply that 'ultimately' regulatory agencies promote the welfare of private industry above other interests because of the prospect of capital accumulation that this offers the state (Jessop 1990). In either case, these interests may be realised within agencies by the threat of legislative oversight or, more significantly, by the executive's power of appointment and removal of senior regulators. According to Majone (1996: 38), in the US, executive presidential control is often more direct than Congressional oversight. In five out of seven American regulatory agencies examined in the 1980s, the most effective tool of executive political control was the power to appoint – agency outputs shifted immediately after a change in leadership. Under these circumstances, the corporatist regulatory state exchanges influence on policy development for industrial conduct and control which are consistent with the agencies' interests.

Other options include institutional expansion, competition with other regulatory agencies and the career ambitions of regulators. Over time, the bargaining position of regulators becomes stronger as they accumulate technical and institutional expertise, giving them more autonomy for self-interested projects. For instance, a corporatist regulatory state, whose interests include expansionism, is likely to adopt a bargaining position which maximises its resource allocation subject to the constraints of its other institutional interests. Of course, the precise nature of the agency's

bargaining position depends on the balance of interests determining resource allocation (e.g. the legislature, government
ministers or private industry). As for senior regulators with ambi-
tious career expectations, they may aim to make their agency
more highly regarded by its political and clientele environment
than other agencies:

> Their political instincts are even more sensitive since they are
> anxious to get ahead in the world. They must build or main-
> tain a reputation, and at the same time they must not make
> too many enemies. Generally speaking, they walk this line by
> being 'efficient'.
>
> (Owen and Braeutigam 1978: 2–3)

In short, the nature of agencies' bargaining and negotiation
over policy matters depends on the norms of the particular polity,
including those of regulators themselves.

Some commentators have introduced the idea of a hybrid regulatory state, which exhibits some aspects of pluralism and some
aspects of corporatism. For example, Atkinson and Coleman
(1985) and Lexchin (1990) refer to 'sponsor pluralism' and 'clientele pluralism' respectively to refer to a policy network
characterised by social closure in which the state abdicates its
authority in certain limited policy areas to a single, narrowly
specialised producer group, while there is an absence of a 'strong
state' capable of exacting promises from the producer group's
members. Sponsor pluralism is similar to corporatism because the
state relinquishes some of its authority to private interests, who in
turn pursue policies with which regulatory officials are in broad
agreement. Like corporatism, industry and regulators become co-
responsible for policy development and implementation in sponsor
pluralism. Thus, unlike the pressure group pluralism of private
interest theorists, industry is not on the outside of the regulatory
process. Sponsor pluralism differs from corporatism because it
implies that the state is not autonomous and regulates from a relatively weak bargaining position.

Some European theorists, focusing on 'political culture', have
challenged the dichotomy between public and private interests,
which they see as a peculiarly American product, especially
capture theory. This critique of the public–private interest dichotomy, and of capture theory in particular, is complex, but may be

simplified by appreciating that it appears in three forms, which we shall refer to as the 'weak-analytic', the 'strong-analytic' and the 'anti-essentialist'. Since Hancher and Moran (1989a; 1989b) put forward all three, apparently as a single holistic perspective, it is sufficient to examine their arguments in this regard.

Of these three positions, the weak-analytic is the least controversial and, in our view, the most reasonable. Supporters of this position acknowledge that regulatory processes differ across geographical space (and time), despite similar economic landscapes and interest group configurations. From this, it is reasonably deduced that, in addition to economic interests, other important factors need to be taken into account to explain regulatory processes. Collectively, those other factors are referred to as 'political culture', which may include: the timing of regulatory developments within specific geographical boundaries; the particular national features of the courts, the legislature or an industry; and more broadly the extent of trust invested in government by a population. As Hancher and Moran explain, ' "Culture" signals an interest in the recurrent tension between the common structural forces shaping regulation in the economies of developed market nations, and the idiosyncrasies introduced by unique historical, national and industrial settings' (1989a: 4).

Thus, attention may need to be paid to political culture in reaching appropriate definitions of private and public interest because 'different national traditions conceive of the public-private authority in different ways and different national traditions allow access to regulatory space to different constellations of actors' (Hancher and Moran 1989b: 280).

The stronger analytical perspective, invoking political culture, holds that the distinction between private interests on the one hand and the public interest on the other is of little or no value in analysing regulation. On this view, 'conventional divisions between public and private spheres of power lose most meaning in regulatory arenas', there is 'little to be gained by depicting the relationship in the dichotomous language of public versus private interests' and 'the language of regulatory capture is largely devoid of meaning' because:

> Regulation under advanced capitalism is best conceived as an activity occurring in economies where the public and private are characteristically mixed, where the dominant actors are powerful

and sophisticated organisations, and where the biggest firms have taken on many features of governing institutions ... 'Public' bodies, like departments of state, routinely represent 'private' interests in the debates surrounding regulation. Formally, private bodies, like trade associations, routinely carry out nominally public roles, such as implementation of particular regulations.

(Hancher and Moran 1989a: 5; 1989b: 276)

This position easily slides into the anti-essentialist view that one should not search for ideals for regulation, let alone the ideal to protect the public interest. It is argued that the purpose of regulation cannot be distorted by the influence of private interests because it is 'unhelpful' to identify or defend 'a clearly delimited sphere of public authority' in the first place (Hancher and Moran 1989b: 274). For these authors, the roles of 'public' and 'private' in the regulatory process cannot be authoritatively distinguished.

There are certainly many instances in regulation when private interests and the public interest coincide. For example, when the FDA stopped the American producers of thalidomide from marketing it in the US, the regulatory agency protected public health and prevented the pharmaceutical firm from going out of business through the crippling lawsuits which would have followed widespread use of the drug by women in the US (Braithwaite 1986: 298). Large private firms may also implement regulations in the public interest. In the pharmaceutical sector, manufacturing firms collect reports of adverse reactions to their drugs and submit them to regulatory agencies. As Hancher and Moran note, some firms or trade associations may be accorded 'public status' with regard to some functions within the regulatory process – self-policing of product advertising, for instance. However, such phenomena do not imply that the distinction between private interests and the public interest should be entirely dissolved. Nor do they imply that some policy objectives cannot be, in principle, identified as serving primarily or wholly private interests as distinct from the public interest, or vice versa. Indeed, reference to the 'public' status of 'formally private' organisations suggests that the public–private conceptual distinction is indispensable.

It follows from this that a basic distinction between public and private interest remains valid, but the precise nature of the distinction is partly dependent on how 'the public interest' and 'private interests' are defined at the outset, and partly dependent on empirical findings. In our view, conceptual problems can be minimised by referring to consumers' interests or patients' interests, rather than 'the public interest'. Whether these interests are coincident with, convergent with, divergent with or in conflict with the interests of private industry is an empirical question, but we cannot even raise the question if the conceptual distinctions are dissolved. As a corollary, it is possible, and arguably helpful, to define 'essentialist' regulatory goals, which are in consumers' interests, and to examine whether or not those goals may be distorted in practice by the influence of private interests or otherwise.

Ironically, as political theorists concentrated on the distinctiveness of European regulation and on the international differences of political culture within Europe, in the 1980s regulatory processes in Europe became more similar to American regulation in two significant respects: 'inter-state' harmonisation, albeit within a supranational rather than federal state; and neo-liberal 'deregulation' and/or 're-regulation'. EU legislation made under the authority of the founding treaties between Member States takes precedence over domestic law in Member States, and passes directly into domestic law. Consequently, a lot of regulation in European countries is increasingly homogenised in response to EU directives. For example, in 1970 about 25 directives and 600 regulations were issued by the Brussels authorities, but by the early 1990s these figures had risen to 80 directives and 1,500 regulations – more legislation than was issued by the French national authorities in 1991 (Majone 1996: 56–9).

EU legislation has not simply replaced national regulations: it has also created new regulatory responsibilities via supranational initiatives from the European Commission. Of particular significance is the phenomenon of harmonisation and the associated re-regulation of product standards at the supranational level, such as harmonisation of regulation between Member States. Harmonisation is the most direct and deliberate strategy for extinguishing international differences in regulation within the EU, irrespective of national political culture. It involves complex procedures and mechanisms of mutual recognition of regulatory judgements together with the development of semi-autonomous supranational regulatory agencies under the auspices of the Commission (e.g. the European Agency for the Evaluation of Medicinal Products).

As Montanari (1995) argues, harmonisation needs to be understood in terms of the EU's fundamental objective in the Treaty of
Rome to create a single European market, and in relation to the
internationalisation of economic interests (Greenwood and Ronit
1991). The latter is important because, as Hancher and Moran
(1989a) emphasise, the operation of transnational firms within the
European regulatory process is pervasive. These firms often seek to
minimise differences in regulations between Member States to avoid
the additional costs of meeting many inconsistent regulatory standards. While distinctive national contexts may continue to affect the
operation of businesses, it is difficult to see how these processes of
Europeanisation cannot undermine the importance of national
political culture within regulation (Lewin 1994; Whitley 1992).

These processes of Europeanisation are analogous, though not
identical, to American developments about a century earlier,
beginning with federal regulation signalled by the Interstate
Commerce Act of 1887. For example, in the US during the nineteenth century, the pharmaceutical trade was regulated solely
within fifty different 'states' (Texas, Pennsylvania, etc.), if at all.
The quality and supply of drugs could differ dramatically from
one 'state' to another. The first federal law regulating the quality
of pharmaceuticals involved in *inter*-'state' commerce within
the US was the 1906 Federal Pure Food and Drug Act – anti-
adulteration legislation. For the first time pharmaceuticals had to
meet the same standards of quality across different 'states'. This
harmonising trend consolidated as the twentieth century
progressed: in 1927, the FDA, a *federal* drug regulatory agency,
was established. Then, as now, it formed a unitary political entity
regulating medicines across all the 'states'. Similar trends occurred
across other sectors of the economy, making up the American
regulatory state. As Majone (1996: 55) argues, by analogy
Europeanisation processes of the last few decades may be regarded
as the development of a 'European regulatory state'.

Whether the European regulatory state advances further towards
an American-style federal state remains to be seen. According to
neo-functionalist theories of international integration that outcome
is to be expected, because they suppose that governmental functions
steadily migrate from the national level to global technocrats
under the impetus of transnational interests seeking to transfer
policy competence to a supranational body (Haas 1958; 1961;
Lindberg 1963). Apart from wishing to avoid inconsistencies in

national regulatory standards, transnational firms may also favour supranational European regulation to prevent progressively more stringent regulations in some of the more zealous Member States. It is not only transnational economic interests which may favour the growth of supranational regulation. Nation-states may also do so in some respects. For example, a Member State, say Germany, might support greater environmental regulation at the EU level, which would be closer to German national controls, because it would minimise administrative costs to the German state and offer a competitive advantage to German industry already familiar with the new regulatory regime (Boehmer-Christiansen and Skea 1991; Majone 1996: 68). The success of this strategy would be determined, in part, by the relative influence of the Member States, which varies with sectors of the economy (Heritier 1996). Furthermore, as we mentioned in our discussion of national agencies, regulatory agencies may also have their own interests in terms of credibility, growth and security. It is reasonable to suppose that EU institutions may also possess such features, adding to the impetus for increased supranational regulatory activity.

The other influence which brought American and European regulatory approaches closer during the 1980s and 1990s was neo-liberalism. As Boreus (1997) notes, two distinct aspects of the neo-liberal perspective are that the state should be minimal and subject to the tests of 'the market'. Often the adoption of this perspective by Western governments entailed deregulation or re-regulation with a 'lighter touch'. Ayres and Braithwaite (1992) caution against assuming that the Reaganite rhetoric of deregulation actually delivered deregulation because of opposition from a Democratic Congress. Nevertheless, the influence of neo-liberal conceptions of the state on governments in this period is unmistakable, especially in many European countries.

On the face of it, there seems to be a considerable tension between the neo-liberal goal of a minimalist state and the growth of EU regulations and supranational regulatory institutions. On the other hand, the harmonisation of trade into a single European market should be seen in the context of the European Single Market Programme of the mid-1980s, which developed as a response to the perceived economic decline of Europe relative to Japan and the United States in the world economy (Wyatt-Walter 1995). Since the mid-1980s a key element in the drive for a single European market has been market liberalisation (Begg 1996).

Paradoxically, it may be that a strong regulatory state is needed to impose marketisation (Wilks 1996). However, the interaction between Europeanisation of regulation and neo-liberal influences on the state remains to be more fully theorised.

## Technical expertise, regulatory science and citizenship

Regulatory agencies handle specialised areas of socioeconomic activity. Their attraction to politicians is that they develop expertise and a continuity of concern over a set of problems. Generalist politicians in the legislature and the executive do not have the knowledge, time or inclination to foster such expertise. Moreover, an important source of legitimation for regulatory agencies is often that technical expertise can be a motor for social progress, unsullied by the influences of party politics. In short, while elected politicians in the executive appoint senior regulators, the bulk of regulatory decision-making is delegated to regulatory agencies.

The growth of regulatory agencies in Western Europe and North America over the last century means that an increasing part of government in these liberal democracies is conducted by technical experts, who are unelected. This is especially so because of governments' belief that science and technology are of central importance for economic growth, associated with large-scale technological complexity and rapid rates of economic and technological change. Indeed, even during the course of judicial reviews of agencies' conduct, the courts are very reluctant to challenge any regulatory judgements that might be regarded as 'technical', preferring to defer to the agencies' expertise on such matters (Kendall 1991). This raises questions about the democratic accountability and credibility of regulatory agencies – questions that are potentially more acute for supranational regulatory institutions in the EU because their links with citizens are more contorted and obscure than their national counterparts. Both the legitimatory demand for technical expertise and the problem of democratic accountability are magnified many times when the products being regulated are science-based – as in the regulation of medicines, pesticides, genetically modified food, industrial chemicals, nuclear power plants and so on and so forth. So pervasive is the role of scientific experts in such regulatory policy-making that Jasanoff (1990) regards them as another branch of government.

Typically, in controlling science-based products, technical experts in regulatory agencies, drawing on the expertise of external scientific advisors, make assessments about the risks and benefits of the new products for the purposes of policy-making. This process, known as 'regulatory science' (or 'mandated science'), is less concerned with discovery and new knowledge, as validated by peers in refereed journals, than academic research science (Jasanoff 1990: 76–8; Weinberg 1972). Rather, regulatory science involves studies commissioned by government officials to aid decision-making and the review and evaluation of published research, which may be useful for regulation. Thus, meta-analysis and evaluation of the scientific literature is often the end-product in regulatory science, while in academic science it is usually the first step in a research programme (Salter 1988).

Regulatory science includes 'knowledge production designed to fill gaps in the knowledge base relevant to regulation', 'knowledge synthesis' refocused on matters of regulatory significance, and 'prediction' of the likely risks or benefits of the new science-based technology (Jasanoff 1990: 77). However, because of the heavy influence of industry in the production of science-based products, whose development and success partly depend on meeting regulatory standards, regulatory science should also be seen as including the industrial scientific practices specifically geared to regulatory requirements. As Irwin et al. (1997) emphasise, industry's development and validation of regulatory testing and in-house risk-benefit assessment in preparation for submission to government regulatory agencies are also part of regulatory science.

For some commentators, the implication of regulatory science is that political decisions about risks in society are increasingly forged and dominated by elite networks of scientists in industry, government and industry-funded academic experts. On this view, democracy is giving way to technocracy, which Fischer (1990: 17–18) defines as follows:

Technocracy refers to a system of governance in which technically trained experts rule by virtue of their specialised knowledge and position in dominant political and economic institutions ... But technocracy is more than expertise per se. Expertise can be organised to serve a variety of social functions and interests. Technocracy refers to the adaptation of expertise to the task of governance. It gives rise to a theory of governmental decision making designed to promote technical solutions to political problems.

Critics of technocracy do not suggest that advanced industrialised countries are currently ruled by technocrats. Rather, reminiscent of aspects of corporatist and Marxist theory, the ruling 'class' or 'echelon' of society consists of a 'partnership' of political and economic elites in the executive arm of government and in big business. While technocrats occupy a privileged position in government and other powerful institutions relative to the 'mass public', they receive their rewards, it is argued, from the ruling echelon to whom they give their allegiance as a result (Barnes 1985: 90–112; Offe 1973). A significant consequence, argue theorists of technocracy, is that a key role for technocrats is to shield elites in the ruling echelon from political pressure from 'below' by rendering information inaccessible to the public through technical encoding or norms of 'confidentiality' (Fischer 1990: 27–9). More subtly, expert science advisers within regulatory processes may shift the official boundaries between 'science' and 'politics' ('non-science') according to the policy context in which they are operating (Gieryn 1983; Jasanoff 1987). Thus, regulatory science is regarded as heavily context-dependent, rather than adhering to the universalistic norms of science idealised by writers such as Merton (1942).

According to Fischer (1990), technocrats are sceptical of politics, fundamentally unsympathetic to the openness and equality of political democracy, reject 'moralistic criteria', and are strongly committed to 'technological progress and material productivity', but are less concerned about the distribution of progress and 'social justice'. In particular, he suggests that social debate about the needs for and direction of technological developments becomes marginalised: 'As instrumental techniques replace political substance, the means of policy become the ends. In the process, the essential political question – production for what? – is at best relegated to secondary status. At worst, it is simply ignored' (Fischer 1990: 25).

In arguing for greater citizen participation in regulatory science, Irwin (1995) identifies similar problems with technocratic approaches to environmental risk. He draws attention to the need for a critical debate about the role of science and 'technological culture', which is open to ways of living which are less technologically determined, and calls for a 'more even balance between scientific expertise and the needs of citizens' (Irwin 1995: 4–7, 39–40). According to this perspective, the challenge of regulation and indeed regulatory science is social and political as well as technical, because it raises questions about how we organise our lives and the limits of our control over them. A parallel to this argument in the pharmaceutical sector may be the allegations that there is an overproduction of new drugs which meet little or no therapeutic needs for patients while there is a dearth of research into medicines for rare diseases, and a relative absence of debate about how societies, and health services in particular, might promote and support lifestyles less dependent on medications (Breggin 1993; Chetley 1990, 1995).

While Irwin (1995) sees science as 'flexible' in the face of public scepticism about expert pronouncements on risk, Fischer (1990) is more pessimistic, maintaining that, in technocratic institutions, democracy is taken to be an inappropriate and inferior decision-making system, and that as societies become more technocratic there is likely to be increasing tension between experts and lay persons. Accompanying this trend, there may be an experience of technology as apparently inevitable (Irwin 1995: 2–3). To paraphrase Wright Mills (1959), citizens may feel they are living in a time of big decisions, but they know they are not making any.

Nevertheless, it would be wrong to draw clear-cut distinctions between powerful, elitist, scientific experts, on the one hand, and passive lay people, on the other (as Irwin and Fischer appreciate). Nor should these groups be seen as homogeneous, even in terms of ostensibly scientific matters in regulatory affairs. For example, Gabe and Bury (1996) document the 'fracturing of expert authority' over the safety of the tranquillising drugs known as benzodiazepines. For nearly twenty years some psychopharmacologists had warned of the dangers of the 'tranquillisation of society' – the overusing and overprescribing of these drugs and concomitant risks of dependence (addiction). Meanwhile, expert scientists in pharmaceutical companies and regulatory agencies attested to their safety on the basis of controlled clinical trial data.

Even more challenging for the regulatory science of medicine, expert scientists have bitterly disputed the appropriate methods for clinically testing the efficacy of anti-cancer 'treatments'. Some medical experts have argued that short-term controlled clinical trials which measure effectiveness primarily in terms of tumour shrinkage are not always appropriate, while their opponents uphold this orthodox method of evaluation and question the ethics of long-term controlled clinical trials with cancer patients. Such disputes have, in effect, paralysed the norms of risk-benefit assessment in some cases, such as the claims that vitamin C contains anti-cancer qualities (Richards 1991). Controversies of this kind severely undermine the technocratic view of regulatory science – a point not lost on the advocates of 'citizen science':

> Despite the rhetoric to the contrary, scientific analyses must reflect the ideological and institutional assumptions of the experts who conduct them – although these assumptions are not necessarily consciously made and indeed their existence may be strongly denied by those who hold them.
>
> (Irwin 1995: 30)

Moreover, 'social movements', including consumer organisations, environmental organisations and public health advocacy groups, often employ or recruit their own scientific experts, who may utilise scientific analyses in order to criticise the regulatory regime hitherto accepted by mainstream scientists in government and industry. This 'scientization of the protest against science' implies that different institutional contexts can foster not only experts with varying ideological predispositions, but also different scientific knowledge about technological risks and benefits (Beck 1992: 161).

A more spectacular aspect of such scientisation, much closer to the concept of 'citizen science', is when lay people become 'experts'. This occurred when some people in the US who were found to be HIV positive or suffering from AIDS organised into a highly effective pressure group, known as the AIDS Coalition To Unleash Power (ACT UP) – similar groups formed in Europe. ACT UP not only campaigned for development of preventative and curative treatments for AIDS, they became directly involved in analysing and debating the regulatory science of drug testing, challenging the traditional separation of testing and treatment. They argued for faster access to experimental anti-AIDS drugs and faster approval for anti-AIDS drugs which had completed clinical testing. For members of ACT UP, the fact that a potential therapy is not proven by the canons of 'good science' should not mean that access is restricted when no effective alternatives exist to treat a life-threatening disease. This brought them into direct confrontation with drug regulatory agencies, such as the FDA, and sections of the medical profession, whose expertise defined whether the risk-benefit ratio of a new drug was acceptable for patients (Epstein 1996; 1997). Initially at least, an unlikely alliance between industry arguments for deregulation and ACT UP's citizen science emerged:

> In fact, large parts of the AIDS advocates' critique of the FDA could have been scripted by the Pharmaceutical Manufacturers' Association. Governments must act faster, tell manufacturers precisely what it wants to know, and let consumers and their physicians decide what risks they want to run. Do not worry so much about a few injuries. Do not dally to conduct more tests on animals. When death is the alternative, get on with the job of finding good therapies.
> (Edgar and Rothman 1990: 124)

The ACT UP campaigns of the 1980s altered the regulatory science of new drugs at the FDA. Much more permissive new criteria for the approval of drugs directed to an immediately life-threatening disease have been introduced, and since 1988 the FDA has been encouraged to become involved with manufacturers in the planning of clinical trials. Specifically, if a manufacturer plans to test drugs to treat life-threatening illnesses, then scientists at the firm may meet with FDA officials early in the development process to reach agreement on the design of the necessary clinical and pre-clinical studies (Edgar and Rothman 1990). The onus to develop anti-AIDS drugs shifted clearly to industry, which became the target of the ACT UP campaigns in the 1990s.

Experiences such as these have encouraged theorists of 'citizen science' (or 'technological citizenship') to argue that highly technical policy decisions need not be exceptions to democratic practice, and that regulatory agencies should be more pro-active in making provisions for citizen participation in risk-benefit assessments of technologies. This position is not based solely on the view that democratic policy-making is morally preferable to alternatives, but also on the belief that lay knowledge, which is currently excluded on the grounds of irrationality, might enrich decision-making processes. The improved communication effected by organising lay people into the expert systems of specialists and confronting specialists with lay experiences might make regulation more workable (Kendall 1991; Vaughan 1989). As Wynne (1980) appreciates, greater citizen participation is likely to be facilitated by a reduction in the secrecy that surrounds the work of many agencies, and he further laments the resistance in science to exploring whether 'embedded levels of standardisation, certainty or other commitments might need to be renegotiated' (Wynne 1995: 385).

According to Fiorino (1990), democratic public participation enables citizens to define issues, question technical experts, dispute evidence and shape the regulatory agenda. Just as the members of ACT UP learned about the medical science of HIV and the testing of anti-AIDS drugs, it is envisaged that citizens acquire their own expertise in the course of involvement in the regulatory process (e.g. in 'citizen review panels'). Indeed, some theorists see such learning as an obligation of 'technological citizenship', along with lay participants' obligations to maintain vigilance and scepticism towards new technologies (Frankenfield 1992). As Laird (1993: 354–5) puts it:

> Participants need to learn from experts but also to understand that experts often disagree with each other and that their advice is usually a complex mixture of facts and values. It is important that participants retain for themselves the analytical prerogatives of determining what questions to ask and how to ask them. They should not simply acquire information from experts.

In addition, some lay knowledge can be generated entirely independently of experts. Often referred to as 'popular epidemiology', this is 'the process whereby lay persons gather scientific data and other information' in order to understand the occurrence of hazards and disease (Brown 1987, 1992: 269; Williams and Popay 1994). In popular epidemiology, it is argued, untrained citizens offer valid perspectives on technical issues, which may produce 'creative conflict' with the epidemiological research of established experts (Irwin 1995: 172). Thus, Funtowicz and Ravetz (1993: 740) propose that citizens involved in popular epidemiology, who are usually directly affected by the risks and benefits of a new technology, can 'perform a function analogous to that of professional colleagues in the peer review or refereeing process in traditional science'. Under these conditions, citizen science is located at the heart of knowledge production within regulatory science.

It is implicit and sometimes explicit in the arguments put forward by advocates of citizen science that direct public participation is desirable because it enhances democracy and regulatory decision-making in terms of promoting public health. However, Perhac (1998) suggests that the issues to be confronted in democratising regulatory science are more complex than critics of technocracy imply. He argues that democracy should not be reduced to public participation or public opinion because it also has a 'constitutional' dimension, which limits the legitimate scope of the influence of public sentiment. For example, the constitutional right to free speech in democracies cannot be legitimately denied as a result of public pressure. Perhac poses the problem that the cost of greater citizen participation and consequent political viability might be 'scientific rigour or the protection of public health', and concludes:

> There may be principles or values, such as the protection of public health, that should not be subject to the test of public under-standing, public perceptions, or majority or special interest values ... The task, then, is to determine which principles or values are so fundamental that they should be embodied regardless of public sentiment, and which are more appropriately treated as prefer-ences that should be put to the test of public sentiment.
>
> (Perhac 1998: 238)

The 'constitutionalist' and 'citizen science' perspectives are not necessarily mutually exclusive. Those subscribing to the latter probably accept that the protection of public health is a funda-mental principle for democracy, while appreciating that what counts as 'protection of public health' is highly contentious because the evaluation of risks and benefits to public health are sometimes unclear or even in dispute. On the other hand, Perhac reminds us that, whatever the degree and mode of citizen participation in regulatory science, the constitutional purpose of regulatory agen-cies remains an important fundamental reference point. In so doing, there is also a warning against basing 'citizen science' on a judgemental relativism which views scientific disputes and claims to expertise as nothing more than ideological manifestos.

## Scientific uncertainty, drug development and public health

Different social and institutional contexts can lead to different scientific uncertainties and estimates of risk (Carvalho de Mello and Machado de Freitas 1998; Levidow *et al.* 1997). So it is with drug development and testing, which have generated their own kinds of technical uncertainties and relations to public health. In saying this we do not imply that the technical aspects of drug testing are entirely separate from social context but, as Irwin (1995: 28–9) notes, such distinctions can sometimes be useful for analytical purposes. This is especially true for pharmaceuticals, whose conventions for development and testing have become widely standardised.

In deciding whether or not patients should be exposed to a newly developed drug, it is necessary to make some risk-benefit assessment of the prospective medicine in question. To do this, medicines regulators and others turn to a science of drug testing, which comprises pre-clinical pharmacology (including efficacy, metabolic and toxicological assessments in animals), safety studies in healthy human volunteers, clinical trials with patients and a form of epidemiology, known as pharmacovigilance. The most significant aspect of pharmacovigilance is post-marketing surveillance, which tracks patients' adverse experiences with drugs on the market by the collection of spontaneous reports of suspected adverse drug reactions (ADRs) from doctors or manufacturers. These scientific enterprises form an integral part of drug product evaluation procedures within the pharmaceutical industry and the governments that regulate it (Lumley and Walker 1985). In order to market new drugs, pharmaceutical companies have to comply with batteries of safety and efficacy tests set by the appropriate regulatory authorities.

Safety and efficacy testing of drugs is characterised by considerable uncertainties. While a small amount of toxicology is undertaken in governments and universities, the toxicological testing of specific drug products is almost always conducted within the industry. In principle at least, the scientific objective of drug toxicology is to estimate the potential toxicity of pharmaceuticals to humans (Barnes and Denz 1954; World Health Organisation 1969: 15; Zbinden 1987). Toxicologists draw on data derived from *in vitro* studies of cell behaviour carried out in glass dishes and on *in vivo* research conducted with whole live animals. Using these two types of data they try to predict the toxicity of a compound in humans.

General toxicological testing provides information on whether the drug is likely to be widely toxic in a range of species, while special toxicity studies, including carcinogenicity and reproductive studies, help identify specific problems. Some, but not all, toxicological tests on a new drug are pre-clinical: that is, they are completed before clinical testing begins. A new drug is also tested for toxicity in healthy people before being given to patients in clinical trials. The pharmaceutical manufacturers take the lead in organising and conducting clinical testing but, unlike toxicological testing, the industry generally involves the wider medical profession at this stage, especially high-status doctors in academia or teaching hospitals who might be sympathetic to the manufacturers' endeavours. Generally clinical testing takes the form of double-blind controlled clinical trials which provide comparative data about the toxicity and effectiveness of new drugs in patient groups.

Both toxicological tests and controlled clinical trials may continue after a medicine has been put on the market. However, at that stage, data based on spontaneous reports of suspected ADRs experienced by patients, either in general practice or during hospital treatment, becomes available. Pharmacovigilance data, derived from post-marketing surveillance systems, are collected initially by pharmaceutical companies and doctors who may then report them to governmental drug regulatory authorities. Pharmaceutical companies are required by law to report ADRs to various degrees in the UK, US and EU, but the arrangements by which doctors make such reports are voluntary.

In saying that regulators turn to the science of drug testing in order to make risk-benefit assessments and, ultimately, decisions about whether to approve new drugs, it is important to appreciate the interaction between the science and politics of medicines regulation. To a large extent, pharmaceutical companies carry out such testing in order to meet the technical standards demanded of them by the regulatory authorities empowered to permit or withhold licence to market. In this sense, the regulatory science of drug testing has developed pragmatically to adjust to shifts in policy (Brown 1988; Lumley and Walker 1985; Schwartzmann 1976).

Moreover, a recurring feature of medicines regulation is that the underpinning science is characterised by considerable technical uncertainty. In toxicology, problems concerning the extrapolative validity of animal and cell studies to humans are substantial. On reviewing the pharmacology of six drugs in humans, dogs and rats, Litchfield concluded that 'many of the most serious side-effects that can result when a drug is given to man were not predictable from observations on dogs or rats' (1961: 34). Optimistically, pre-clinical tests are estimated to have a predictive value of only 65–70 per cent (Rawlins 1994: 34–5).

In the case of testing whether a compound causes cell mutation, *in vitro* mutagenicity tests are employed, but these frequently yield inconsistent results and cannot, for example, determine whether a compound might induce cancer, because only some cancers develop by genetic mechanisms (World Health Organisation 1974: 8–9). For these reasons, it is supposed that *in vivo* lifetime toxicity tests with whole live animals are required to detect carcinogenic (i.e. cancer-inducing) compounds. Salsburg (1983) provided a fairly comprehensive quantitative estimate of the validity of life-time feeding studies of chemicals with rodents as tests for carcinogenicity, and determined that they were more often wrong than right. While there may have been an improvement in the predictive value of animal carcinogenicity studies in the 1990s, such fundamental uncertainties in toxicology have not been over-come (Abraham and Reed 1998).

Of course, with clinical trials there is no problem of extrapolation between species because drugs are administered to humans in such testing. However, only a small sample of the prospective population to be exposed to the drug can be studied in clinical trials. In the UK, for example, the number of patients exposed to a new drug prior to approval is on average about 1,500, although the actual number can vary considerably depending on the product (Rawlins 1994). This is sufficient to detect with confidence only those adverse drug reactions (ADRs) occurring with an incidence of 1 in 500 or greater, assuming zero background incidence. In addition, at the time of marketing, it is rare for more than 100 patients to have received the product for a year or more (Rawlins *et al.* 1992).

Furthermore, patients enrolling in clinical trials usually repre-sent a selected and relatively homogeneous population, whereas a more heterogeneous patient group is likely to receive the drug during general use. Certain kinds of patients who will probably be exposed to the drug if marketed may be excluded from clinical trials because their multiplicity of ill-health or the other medica-tions they are taking might interfere with the scientific demands of controlled comparison (Holford 1995). As Burley and Glynne put it: 'a great deal of artificial rigidity has necessarily to be built in [to clinical trials] which is at odds with normal clinical practice' (1985: 104). As a result, extrapolating findings about the safety and efficacy of medicines from clinical trials to the entire patient population is problematic. There may also be ethical reasons for such uncertainty. For example, it may be considered unethical to treat cancer or AIDS patients for very long on a new but toxic drug that has yet to prove its efficacy relative to other treatments available.

One indicator of the scale of the problem and the effectiveness of pre-marketing evaluation is provided by the number of drugs withdrawn after marketing. However, accurate information on the actual rate of drug withdrawals is hard to come by. According to CSM figures, between 400 and 500 new drugs, called new active substances (NASs), have been approved in the UK since modern controls were introduced in 1972.[1] Of these, some 15 (3–4 per cent) have been withdrawn for safety reasons (Rawlins 1993). From 1961 to 1995, safety-related problems led to the withdrawal of almost a hundred drug products in Germany, France, the UK, the US and Sweden (Darbourne 1995). In addition to outright withdrawals, there have been several other major safety issues, such as the effects of benzodiazapines and oral contraceptives, the contamination of blood products and the link between human pituitary extracts and Creutzfeldt–Jakob disease. All these examples testify to the difficulties involved in predicting adverse reactions.

As regards the pharmacovigilance data collected after medicines are on the market, the difficulties are less about extrapolation and more about interpretative uncertainty. The collection of ADR data as a planned activity has been undertaken for about thirty years (Alvarez-Requejo and Porta 1995; Lawson 1984). Some commentators divide pharmacovigilance methods into two types: the informal spontaneous reporting of ADRs by doctors, which remains by far the most important aspect of pharmacovigilance in medicines regulation; and the formal collection of epidemiological data (Rawlins et al. 1992; Rawlins 1993).

The fact that the spontaneous reporting of ADRs by doctors is voluntary means that the proportion of real ADRs such reports represent for any particular product is unknown, although in general terms it is thought that doctors in the UK report about 5–10 per cent of such reactions (Walker and Lumley 1987). Nevertheless, such reporting is also thought to vary over time in ways that are not necessarily predictable. In the UK such reporting was falling in the late 1990s, while supplementary ADR collection systems have also withered (Anon 1997i). Interpretation also relies on reliable estimates of the size and demographic features of the exposed population – the so-called 'denominator problem' in the calculation of relative risk. Surrogate measures, such as prescription information and sales data, offer a crude estimate but do not provide sufficiently accurate information for the optimal use of data (Rawlins 1993).

These problems mean that any attempt to make quantitative comparisons between the ADRs reported for different drugs is characterised by substantial uncertainty. To compound these difficulties, the nature of the reports themselves indicates association but not necessarily causation between the drug product and adverse reaction. The doctor may suspect that the drug caused the reaction, but may not have established this. In the context of normal clinical practice, patients may be suffering from many illnesses and be taking many drugs in addition to the one under suspicion (Inman 1986). Under these conditions it is generally much more difficult to establish a causal link between a drug and adverse reaction than it is during clinical trials (Mann 1987). Ideally, recognition of the 'signals' of risk provided by reporting schemes would be based on high-quality information on background incidence rates, but this is often lacking. Despite its importance, spontaneous reporting therefore has serious limitations.

Formal pharmacovigilance methods include scrutiny of vital statistics, case registries, case control (cross-sectional) studies and cohort (longitudinal) studies, all of which may be regarded as types of epidemiological studies. While these methods solve the 'denominator problem', the population under consideration is much smaller than that in spontaneous reporting schemes, though larger than in clinical trials. But unlike most controlled clinical trials, epidemiological studies are observational and hence potentially subject to biases and confounding factors. Also, such epidemiological studies tend to be long and complicated, whereas spontaneous reporting schemes provide much more rapid information in face of the need to make a regulatory decision about a potentially dangerous drug on the market. Hence, the extent to which formal and informal pharmacovigilance provides valid and reliable data upon which regulatory authorities and others can reach assessments about medicines safety is also limited.

To compound the technical uncertainties underpinning medicines regulation, the three data sets, toxicology, clinical trials and pharmacovigilance, may not produce consistent and confirmatory results, and indeed different scientific standards may be applied as to how consistencies between these very different types of data should be defined (Abraham and Sheppard 1998). There is often also the problem of balancing the (possible or probable) harm caused to some patients against the potential benefits to others. In this sense, drug regulatory decisions are specific examples of the more general socio-political problem: namely, how societies decide on 'acceptable' levels of risk from a particular hazard. These deep and extensive uncertainties in drug testing partly account for the fact that scientists in different national regulatory authorities can review the same data about the safety of a medicine and reach entirely contradictory regulatory decisions about it (Abraham 1995). However, as we have indicated, such uncertainties do not exist in a social or economic vacuum. Fundamentally, pharmaceutical companies have real commercial interests in getting their drug products marketed quickly, while patients have real health interests in receiving medicines that they need and that are maximally safe and effective. Sometimes these interests converge, but in other instances they may diverge or even conflict.

Pharmaceutical companies need research and development (R and D) in order for new drug products to be developed. The discovery and development of a NAS is a time-consuming and expensive task. Many research efforts fail because the compounds discovered do not demonstrate any therapeutic value. Allowing for failures, the cost of bringing a NAS to the market may be £100–200 million. Successful R and D needs to meet the overlapping criteria defined by market competition and regulation. To be of value to its manufacturer, a new drug product must be attractive to doctors and/or consumers compared with other drugs on the market, while also meeting regulatory requirements of quality, safety and therapeutic efficacy in order to be permitted on the market.

Typically, at least 50 per cent of R and D spending represents the costs of animal and clinical testing (Burstall 1990: 16). For prescription drugs, which make up between 80 and 95 per cent of the market in different EU countries, persuading doctors to prescribe them is crucial to their commercial success. A new drug will be profitable to its manufacturer if it gains marketing approval and commands a sufficiently large market long enough to more than recover its R and D costs. On the other hand, if the R and D costs of a drug are very high and its potential market is relatively low, then that product may make a loss or, perhaps more likely, may be abandoned during development because its lack of profitability is foreseen by the company.

To add to the complexity, the nature of the market, and indeed market competition, is shaped by laws about intellectual property rights. When a research-based company discovers a NAS, it can prevent any competitor from exploiting the discovery by taking out a patent. However, patents have a limited life-span of twenty years in the EU. Thereafter, other firms (known as the generics pharmaceutical industry) may 'copy' the compound to produce generic drugs (or 'generics') for their own commercial purposes. Hence, manufacturers have a commercial interest in developing, testing and gaining marketing approval for their NASs quickly so that they can recoup their R and D investments before the patents expire.

One reason why the nature of medicines regulation is enormously important to the pharmaceutical industry is because it affects these commercial aspects of drug development. Stringent regulations may drive up R and D costs because of clinical and toxicological testing requirements, and may also reduce potential time on the market to recoup those costs if the longevity of R and D also needs to be increased to meet regulatory requirements. Similarly, if the regulatory process is relatively slow – that is, if it takes a long time for manufacturers to obtain marketing approval after submitting their applications to regulators – then this may further erode the time on the market before patents expire, and hence profits. This problem for the industry has been partially addressed by an EU Regulation 1768/92, which provides up to fifteen years' protection after marketing authorisation in the EU (Hancher 1996: 182).

Nevertheless, structurally, pharmaceutical manufacturers have a commercial interest in relatively unintrusive regulation and in relatively rapid approval times by regulatory authorities. Successful new drugs may earn US$1 million per day in global sales revenues (Vogel 1998: 7). Clearly, a far-reaching citizen science of medicines regulation could come into conflict with a regulatory science built around commercialised intellectual property rights (Etzkowitz and Webster 1995). This is not to suggest that all individuals who work for pharmaceutical companies do so purely for reasons of commercial gain. Indeed, some scientists in the industry have become 'whistle-blowers' on the actions of their employers, which they believe are contrary to 'the public interest', rather than prioritising commercial secrets (Nelkin 1984).

Moreover, it is clear that firms also have an interest in avoiding drug disasters, which may damage their credibility among the medical profession, adversely impact on share prices, and/or prove costly in drug injury litigation. In these respects, the industry accepts the basic need for regulatory authorities to protect public health, but the appropriate extent of regulatory intervention has been contentious throughout the twentieth century, and remains so. For example, the extent to which drug testing and regulatory checks, which are costly to industry, can be reduced before exposing patients to unacceptable risks or even drug disasters, is not predictable, so it becomes a matter of social negotiation. Thus, not only may socioeconomic and political contexts frame scientific uncertainties, but technical paradigms of drug testing, once established, bear intrinsic uncertainties which usher in social and political judgements on a more or less routine basis under the guise of technical problem-solving.

## Conclusion

The foregoing discussion provides a framework for empirical investigation of European medicines regulation and is highly suggestive of important research questions to be addressed by that investigation. In concluding this chapter, we draw out some of the implications of the above theoretical framework for research on European medicines regulation. In moving from the 'theoretical' to the 'empirical', these take the form of specific problems related to the pharmaceutical sector.

In the EU, most medicines reach patients via their doctors, on prescription. Even doctors (as 'consumers in the market') do not have the resources to scrutinise new drugs for safety and efficacy. In this basic sense, the pharmaceutical market requires a 'regulatory state' to correct its 'information failures'. Whatever the interactions, overlaps and complexities of public and private interests, it is clear that pharmaceutical companies have real commercial interests in maximising profits from their products, and that patients have real health interests in having access to safe medicines that are needed.

Because the transfer of regulatory powers to the EU level has also created new regulatory responsibilities at the national level, the European regulatory state must be understood as a network, including supranational and national bodies. This means that it is important to understand the contexts of national regulatory systems in Europe, for these have shaped – and have been shaped by – Europeanisation processes. But how substantial is

Europeanisation of medicines regulation and the development of a European regulatory state in the pharmaceutical sector, and how should it be characterised? Pluralist? Captured? Consumer protective? Corporatist? Neo-liberal? Democratic or technocratic? For example, bearing in mind Perhac's constitutionalist perspective, how does Europeanised medicines control fit with the World Health Organisation's definition of the basic purpose of drug regulation as 'the need to ensure that in drug matters the prescriber and the patient can be reasonably assured of efficacy, safety, quality and truth' (Dukes 1985: 36)?

In scrutinising transnational pharmaceutical regulation in Europe, it is necessary to consider whether the internationalisation of industrial interests and concomitant European integration might have eroded corporatist tendencies. Insofar as there has been social closure around technical expertise in medicines regulation, has Europeanisation undermined this, thereby releasing new pluralist energies, or has it merely strengthened supranational regulatory bodies at the expense of national regulatory agencies? How is increased Europeanisation affecting national drug regulatory systems?

It is also important to take account of how neo-liberal and corporatist tendencies may be interacting at the national and transnational levels. In particular, has neo-liberalism supplanted corporatism? If so, what role do the legislature and the executive arms of government play in this new political environment? Is European harmonisation of medicines regulation likely to raise or lower the safety standards, and how far are these judgements driven by politics or science? Are European drug regulatory agencies behaving technocratically by neglecting to consider whether drug products are needed in favour of productivity *per se*? How well are they addressing issues of democracy, accountability and citizen participation in medicines regulation, perhaps via public rights of access to government information and transparency of decision-making? How pro-active are they in making provisions for citizen participation in regulatory science? Are the intellectual property rights of pharmaceutical companies being balanced effectively against democratic accountability in the overall interests of public health?

These are some of the key questions we explore in the following chapters, as we probe into the world of the European pharmaceutical industry, its regulators and frequent opponents in consumer interest groups.

# Chapter 2

# Opening the black box of European medicines regulation
## Methodology and terminology

Research on the Europeanisation of medicines regulation must, of course, analyse the appropriate institutions which operate at the level of the EU. However, it is important not to lose sight of national institutions and their development within individual European countries. It is our contention that, in the case of European medicines regulation, it is desirable to examine not merely the transnational EU systems or, say, the UK–EU interface, but also to compare different European countries in order to appreciate the nature of the interaction between European regulation, scientific expertise and public health. The reasons for adopting such an approach are that a national position towards medicines harmonisation may have influenced, and been influenced by, the positions taken by other EU countries; and that explanations of differences and similarities in regulatory priorities and practices across different Member States can provide valuable insights into why harmonisation takes one particular route rather than another. Furthermore, a defining characteristic of the 'Europeanisation' of medicines regulation is that some powers remain with Member States, and the utilisation of those powers can only be examined if some analysis focuses on the national level.

At the end of Chapter 1, we outlined the central and broad research problems motivating our research. During the course of the research, those problems were broken down into much more specific questions about the Europeanisation of medicines regulation. In this chapter, we discuss how the empirical research was designed and the methods used to collect and analyse our data. Finally, we address ourselves to some key terminological matters in order to clarify meaning and improve understanding of the discussions in subsequent chapters.

## Research design

Our research is concerned with *prescription* medicines, rather than over-the-counter drugs. In Europe, prescription medicines are, in general, therapeutically more powerful, potentially more toxic and scientifically more significant than their over-the-counter counterparts. For these reasons they pose more substantial regulatory problems and, as such, constituted a more appropriate field of investigation for our research. This is not to be dismissive of over-the-counter drugs. Undoubtedly, much research on the regulation of those products in Europe remains to be done.

Moreover, primary attention is given to the regulatory process for new drugs (NCEs and NASs) because they are the most significant in terms of an appraisal of changing national and European regulatory standards, and because they are of great significance for public health and regulatory science. Nonetheless, a substantial amount of regulatory activity is concerned with (often minor) variations – that is, any change to an existing drug product on the market – and generic drugs – 'copy-products' produced after the patent has expired on a manufacturer's brand-name medicine. Similarly, our focus is primarily on the research-based pharmaceutical industry. However, it is important to note that generic product manufacturers are also deeply interested in the Europeanisation of medicines regulation. Indeed, considerable debate centres around EU laws on patenting, intellectual property rights and 'market exclusivity' for patent-holders. These are areas which heavily impact on the generics drug industry and, again, this is an area where more fruitful research could be undertaken.

Highly significant changes to European medicines regulation occurred in January 1995 and January 1998 (see Chapters 4–7). Thus, the timing of our research enabled us to compare these 'old' (pre-1995) and new (post-1995) regulatory systems from the perspectives of the major actors involved. Specifically, we investigated the EU's concertation and centralised procedures of drug regulation and the Europeanised procedures of mutual recognition of drug evaluations, involving national and EU bodies (see Chapter 4). Fieldwork for that research took us to the European Commission in Brussels and the European Agency for the Evaluation of Medicinal Products (EMEA) in London. Members of the EMEA's expert decision-making committee were also accessed at appropriate locations within Europe.

At the national level, we decided to focus on Germany, Sweden and the UK. There are several reasons for this choice of 'sample', some of which derive from commonalities and others which are based on contrast. First, and fundamental to all 'sampling', our restrictions on time and resources meant that we could not research all parts of the EU. Second, as our research was concerned with 'science-based' *product* regulation (as distinct from regulation of drug promotion, advertising or pricing) these three countries were chosen because they all have a well-developed research-based pharmaceutical industry (Germany is the largest European exporter of pharmaceutical products, the UK is the home of three of the world's largest pharmaceutical companies and Sweden has a highly developed medical science base, although its pharmaceutical industry is comparatively small in global terms). Third, along with France and the Netherlands, these countries are the leading regulatory authorities in Europe and so potentially the most influential actors in the Europeanisation of medicines regulation. Fourth, their historical relationship to Europeanisation spans the full continuum: Germany has been at the centre of the EU since its inception, the UK was a relative latecomer, and Sweden joined as recently as 1 January 1995. (We wanted to be sensitive to the possibility that the longevity of membership of the European Community might influence the approach taken by national regulatory agencies, and to examine how Europeanisation might affect new members of the EU.) Fifth, as regards government–industry relations, during the 1990s Sweden and the UK have developed regulatory review systems which are funded entirely by fees from the pharmaceutical industry, whereas Germany's regulatory agency continues to receive at least half its funding from taxation. (We wanted to be able to examine whether the retention of state funding for regulatory agencies influenced the approach of regulators.) And sixth, while drug regulation is treated with a very high degree of confidentiality in Germany and the UK, Sweden has a long tradition of 'freedom of information' legislation. (We wanted to examine how the latter would operate in the context of European drug regulation compared with the other more 'secretive' countries.)[1]

## Research methods

Our research began in 1994 and finished in 1999. In broad terms the research was characterised by documentary research supplemented by an extensive programme of interviews conducted in Germany, Sweden, the UK, Brussels and occasionally in other locations in Europe. Most of the documentary research was completed prior to the interview fieldwork, but a considerable amount of documentary data was collected in the field. Key documents reviewed were: medical and pharmaceutical journals, regulatory affairs journals, *Scrip* – the main international trade press of the pharmaceutical industry – the official publications of the European Commission, and the relevant regulatory and technical guidelines/recommendations produced by regulators and industry associations at the relevant national and European levels.

The aim of the interview programme was to find out the views and experiences of industry, regulators and other key groups involved concerning the Europeanisation of medicines regulation. In particular, we sought to: access their perspectives on the relationship between European harmonisation, scientific expertise, public health and 'freedom of information'; gauge their opinions on future developments and expectations of medicines regulation in the EU; and collect first-hand knowledge of the regulatory structures and the challenges confronting each of these groups. A further aim was to develop data sets on 'case-study' drugs which had been reviewed under the Europeanised regulatory procedures (see below).

The vast majority of our interviews were conducted during 1995 and 1996. We interviewed twenty regulators, including senior scientists and administrators: three from the British regulatory authorities, the Medicines Control Agency (MCA); nine from the Swedish regulatory authorities, the Medical Products Agency (MPA); five from the German regulatory authorities, the Bundesinstitut fur Arzneimittel und Medizinprodukte (BfArM); and three operating at different European levels, namely EMEA, the Commission's DGIII (the EU Directive for trade and industry) and the European Parliament. One representative of each of the five relevant industrial trade associations was interviewed, namely: the Association of the British Pharmaceutical Industry (ABPI); the Swedish Pharmaceutical Industry Association, known as Lakesindustrieforeningen (LIF); the association of the German research-based pharmaceutical industry known as Verband Forschender Arzneimittelherstellar e.V. (VFA); the association of smaller German drug manufacturers known as the Bundesverband der

Pharmazeutischen Industrie e.V. (BPI); and the European Federation of Pharmaceutical Industry Associations (EFPIA). Forty-one industrialists from twenty-four individual companies were also interviewed. Broadly speaking, contact was made with two types of industry officials: senior regulatory affairs staff, and senior scientists responsible for drug testing, especially safety assessment. Some industry scientists in charge of pharmacovigilance were also contacted. Twelve companies were British-based, three based in Sweden, six based in Germany and three based in Brussels, but because of the transnational nature of the pharmaceutical industry this does not necessarily mean that that a 'national template' can be imposed on each company. For example, sometimes firms conventionally regarded as 'non-British' were interviewed in their UK bases, and so on and so forth. Recognising that all options for national 'labelling' of transnational companies have limitations, we elected to use a 'national template' defined according to the geographical employment location of the respondent.[2]

This was not a random sample. Rather, we targeted individuals in these organisations who were knowledgeable about European safety evaluation and licensing of medicines, and about regulatory affairs. Thus, the responses reflect informed rather than random opinions.[3] Nevertheless, we believe the sample represents a reasonable cross-section of such opinions within industry and the regulatory agencies in the countries studied. Having said that, we make no claims at all regarding the statistical significance of our findings. Some of the interviews with industry officials and with regulators involved several respondents simultaneously (usually two or three respondents). Consequently, it was not always possible to elicit responses from each individual interviewee.

The response rate was 60 per cent from industry and over 65 per cent from the regulators. However, there were some differences between Germany, Sweden and the UK. Dividing the industry respondents into national affiliations is not entirely straightforward because of the transnational nature of pharmaceutical companies. Nevertheless, according to national location of our fieldwork, industry representatives in Sweden were the most willing to be interviewed (75 per cent) compared with their German and British counterparts, of whom only 63 and 46 per cent, respectively, participated. However, for ease of access, about half those approached in industry were based in the UK, while just over a quarter were based in Germany and about a fifth in

Sweden. A very similar trend in response rates emerged for the regulators: 50 per cent in the UK, 66 per cent in Germany and 70 per cent in Sweden. Ultimately, considerably fewer regulators were approached in the UK than in Sweden because the British regulatory authorities were much less interested in helping and participating in the research than their Swedish counterparts, whose enthusiasm facilitated a greater number of regulatory contacts and respondents. The German regulators were marginally more co-operative and helpful than the British. While equal numbers of regulators were not approached in the three countries, we believe that the main reason for differences in the number of respondents between the countries is reflected in the response rates – that is, willingness to co-operate and participate.

The perspectives of consumer organisations interested in pharmaceuticals issues and European harmonisation were also taken into account. Representatives from the German consumer organisation, Stiftung Warentest, and from the European consumers' organisation, known as BEUC, were also interviewed. We found an absence of consumer/public interest group activity regarding medicines regulation in Sweden. One such organisation simply referred us to the MPA and the other did not reply. As for the UK, we relied on the extensive and recent publications of British consumer organisations, such as the National Consumer Council (NCC). In addition, representatives of the ABPI-funded Centre for Medicines Research (CMR) were interviewed, as were a few appropriate academics in Sweden and Germany and a representative of the World Health Organisation (WHO). All interviews were semi-structured, most were tape-recorded and all respondents were offered anonymity. A list of all the organisations from which staff were interviewed is provided in Appendix 1.

Interviews were employed, rather than questionnaires, because we wanted to question our respondents about why they held particular views about European harmonisation, scientific expertise, drug safety and public health. Even in an interview setting it was not always possible to elicit clear individualised responses on all topics. The interviews were transcribed, systematically coded and, in line with the wishes of the respondents, anonymised.

Regarding specific 'case-study' drugs, we wished to scrutinise independently the trajectory of products submitted to Europeanised regulatory procedures. We made determined efforts to obtain the required data, but with very limited success. Candidate drugs were identified and formal requests for access to toxicological and clinical data were made to the appropriate companies, but all were refused because of industry concerns about confidentiality and transparency. Equally important in preventing detailed study of specific drugs were restrictions imposed by national governments and the EU on the release of information about applications and internal evaluation processes. The national regulatory authorities in Germany and the UK refused all access to information about new drug applications because of secrecy laws. The Swedish MPA did provide such information under its Freedom of the Press Act, but only on condition that we did not divulge the information to a third party! As for the EU regulatory authorities, it took unduly long to obtain even a definitive list of drug products approved via Europeanised procedures, as neither the Commission nor the EMEA could decide whether such a list should be made public, and, if so, whose responsibility it was to provide it. This delay may have been in part due to the pressure of work during a period of considerable upheaval in European regulatory systems, but it also reflected the generally secretive and opaque nature of the pharmaceutical sector. While not a great surprise to us, the difficulty in accessing product information held by companies and regulatory agencies is itself an important finding. The stance of both the EMEA and national regulatory agencies towards the availability of data for research, and other purposes is examined further in Chapters 6 and 7.

## Terminological matters

For the non-specialist, the terminological landscape of medicines regulation may at times appear baffling. The purpose of this section is to ease the reader's passage through the interchangeability of various terms used in the literature on medicines regulation. One reason for the variety of terms used is that EU institutions tend to have introduced new terminology which is frequently different from that used in, say, the UK or the US. Our strategy in this section is simply to 'work through' the drug review process up to marketing, highlighting the pertinent terminology as we go along.

When a pharmaceutical firm seeks to get a new prescription drug product approved for marketing by a regulatory agency, the company makes an application to do so. At this stage the firm may also be referred to as 'the applicant', 'the manufacturer' or 'the sponsor'. The data submitted may be known as 'the new drug application', 'the product licence application' or 'the product dossier'. After regulators have completed their review of the dossier, they produce what is known as 'an assessment report'. Before a drug can be approved by regulators, the conditions of its use must be approved, such as the 'indications' (that is, what it can be used to treat) and 'contraindications' (when it should not be used), as well as appropriate dosage, warnings and many other details.

Prior to approval, the regulators and the applicant agree on a document which summarises all these details and is intended to be consulted by prescribing doctors. In the US, this document is sometimes referred to as 'the label' (meaning the doctor's label). In the UK, it has traditionally been referred to as 'the data sheet'. A similar document is referred to as the 'summary of product characteristics' in the context of EU medicines regulation. Furthermore, since 1995 EU Member States, including the UK, increasingly refer to the 'summary of product characteristics', rather than the 'data sheet'. If the regulators decide that the drug may be approved for use, then this is known as 'new drug approval', 'product licensing', 'marketing authorisation' or 'registration', although under some special circumstances, which are not discussed in this book, it is possible for a drug to receive 'registration' without 'marketing authorisation'. The term favoured by the EU to describe drug approval is 'marketing authorisation'.

# Chapter 3

# National regulation
# in Europe

When considering the control of medicines in Europe, two distinct but related sources of government regulation need to be taken into account: the national legislation and institutions of the Member States; and the supranational bodies and laws of the EU. While the Europeanisation of medicines control has undoubtedly been a supranational and transnational phenomenon, it has been built on existing national systems of drug regulation. This process of Europeanisation did not start from a blank slate; it was partly shaped by the socioeconomic and political contexts of EU nation-states. The historical timing of regulatory developments may also be significant because different European countries may influence each other or even dominate 'regulatory space' (Hancher and Moran 1989b: 284–5). Hence, to understand Europeanisation, we must examine the nature of modern national regulation and how it has come about. This must, of course, go beyond legislation because, as Dukes (1985: 32) notes, the interpretation put upon the law by regulatory agencies and other parties involved is of great significance.

In this chapter, we document the development and experience of national medicines control in Germany, Sweden and the UK, leaving the supranational aspects to Chapters 4 to 7. The evolution of drug regulation in these countries is related to the terrain of consumer, professional and industrial interests, whose influence (or lack of) has been felt differently by governments at different times. Appreciating that organisational status is an important condition of access to 'regulatory space', we begin by examining the key organised interests. The role of the state itself has in no small measure come under scrutiny during developments in regulation, leading to various degrees of intervention in the activities of the pharmaceutical industry and market. In the face of drug disasters, the state's involvement in the protection of public health from unsafe drugs has become a political imperative, brushing shoulders, sometimes in the courts, with the commercial interests of pharmaceutical manufacturers in getting and maintaining more drugs on the market. In this highly commercialised and politicised environment, traditional professional interests of medical scientists, such as autonomy and independence, have been challenged and reinvented. This chapter scrutinises how the balance of these social forces has emerged in regulatory developments at the national level.

## The scale and structure of the pharmaceutical industry

The pharmaceutical industries in Germany, Sweden and the UK are among the ten most research-based in the world, keeping company with Belgium, France, Italy, Japan, Switzerland, the Netherlands and the US. Together, the pharmaceutical industries in these ten countries make up about 70 per cent of the world's pharmaceutical production and exports (Davis 1997: 9). In the UK, the industry conducts a substantial amount of research and development (R and D) and has considerable toxicological facilities for drug testing. There are three major British research-based companies, namely Glaxo Wellcome, Smith Kline Beecham and Zeneca (merged with Astra in 1999 to become Astra Zeneca) – all with toxicological facilities in the UK. Indeed, in the mid-1990s, Glaxo Wellcome was reported to spend about £1,200 million on R and D – more than any other company in the world (Davis 1997: 10). However, many companies in the UK are primarily marketing organisations for firms headquartered elsewhere. Such companies usually maintain a regulatory affairs department responsible for managing applications to market new drug products, but lack the scientific capacity to assess drug safety.

The German pharmaceutical industry is larger than its counterpart in the UK, but more fragmented and diverse. The eight main research-based German companies are Bayer, Boehringer Ingelheim, Boehringer Mannheim, Byk Gulden, E Merck, Hoechst Marion Roussel, Knoll and Schering. These conduct research and safety testing, as do many German subsidiaries of foreign companies. Both Bayer and Hoechst Marion Roussel each spend over £600 million annually on R and D and were in the top ten companies in the world for such expenditure in the 1990s (Davis 1997: 10). There are also hundreds of smaller pharmaceutical companies in Germany. The total number of officially registered drug manufacturers is around 1,200, ranging in size from pharmacies selling products under their own name to about forty transnational firms selling worldwide. Consequently, even the larger companies tend to have a smaller market share in Germany than is typical in other countries, which may partly account for Germany's position as a major exporter of medicines.

By contrast, the Swedish pharmaceutical industry, which is much smaller than that in Germany or the UK, is dominated by two research-based companies: Astra AB (Astra Zeneca since 1999) and Pharmacia AB (Pharmacia-Upjohn since 1995). Astra, noted for its decentralised corporate structure, consists of a series of research companies dedicated to specific therapeutic areas, including Astra Charnwood in the UK, as well as companies involved in production and/or marketing. Each of Astra's research companies has its own regulatory affairs department, which is responsible for preparing documentation for marketing. For example, Astra Hassle employ about forty regulatory affairs staff. While a small amount of toxicological and pharmacological work is conducted by these research companies, the majority is carried out centrally at Astra's toxicology and safety assessment laboratories in Gartuna, where there are about 300 staff (Astra AB 1995). Prior to its merger with Upjohn in 1995, Pharmacia was about the same size as Astra but more centralised, with its main research and production sites at Stockholm and Uppsala. In addition to Astra and Pharmacia, there are several small Swedish companies with research capacity, particularly in the field of biotechnology. However, the vast majority of Swedish companies are marketing arms of foreign-based firms.

In each country in the EU, most pharmaceutical companies belong to a national trade association which represents their interests. In the UK, the Association of the British Pharmaceutical Industry (ABPI) represents more than a hundred companies, both UK-based and subsidiaries of foreign firms. The voting rights of member companies are based on sales. It is considered to be the most effective national pharmaceutical industry association in Europe, especially after successfully steering an intensive lobbying campaign to locate the European Agency for the Evaluation of

Medicinal Products (EMEA) in London. The ABPI operates a series of working parties on all aspects of national and European pharmaceuticals policy, including input into the production of technical guidelines about drug testing and relations with regulatory authorities. For example, it organises joint seminars where staff from the British regulatory agency and industry officials meet to discuss specific topics of concern.

While the ABPI may be taken to broadly represent the interests of the British pharmaceutical industry, those interests are not entirely homogeneous. As the controversy in 1999 over the cost-effectiveness of Glaxo Wellcome's anti-flu drug showed, the British Pharmaceutical Group comprising Glaxo Wellcome and Smith Kline Beecham evidently lobbies governments independently of the ABPI. Furthermore, one senior official at a UK company told us that he always encouraged staff to participate in ABPI activities, but added, 'the ABPI does tend to run in little clubs on certain subjects. A little club gets together and they are the privileged few who know what is going on.'[1]

Some other industry officials in the UK went further. One commented that small companies were disenfranchised within the ABPI – a view confirmed by another who suggested the Association found it difficult to meet the needs of smaller manufacturers, whose agenda differed from that of large companies.[2]

It was tensions between the interests of the large research-based companies and other firms in the German pharmaceutical industry that led to the break-up of the national trade association, Bundesverband der Pharmazeutischen Industrie (BPI). Since the break-up in 1994, the BPI has represented mainly small and medium-sized firms, while the large research-based companies have been represented by the 'break-away' Verband Forschender Arzneimittel-herstellar (VFA). There are about forty research-based companies in the VFA. They supply around 70 per cent of prescription medicines in Germany and account for over 90 per cent of research expenditure in the industry there. While there is some overlap between the two associations (e.g. Knoll belongs to both) and some of BPI's 350 members include companies with research capacity, the BPI membership consists predominantly of smaller German manufacturers.

Such diversity and fragmentation is thought to reduce the effectiveness of the German industry's bargaining capacity. It was for this reason that in 1995 the previously fragmented Swedish pharmaceutical industry merged into a single association, the Lakesindustrieforeningen (LIF). The LIF has sixty-five member companies whose sales constitute about 99 per cent of the Swedish market. Efforts to build a single organisation to represent the interests of the Swedish pharmaceutical industry reflect the view among companies that this is the most effective way for them to have influence on the international stage. This goal was sharpened by Sweden's entry into the EU in 1995 (Anon 1995b).

## Consumers and patients as organised interests

Organisations claiming to represent the interests of consumers and patients fall into three basic but overlapping categories: consumer associations, patient associations and public health advocacy groups. Consumer organisations do not specialise in the field of medicines, but periodically engage with issues of medicines regulation, often concentrating on labelling, pricing and transparency. By contrast, public health advocates focus and campaign on matters concerning the safety and therapeutic value of medicines, including the adequacy of drug regulation, the conduct of pharmaceutical companies in testing, promoting and advertising their products, and public rights of access to information about the risk-benefit assessment of new medicines. Organised around the concerns of people suffering from a particular disease or illness, patient associations are even more focused than public health advocates. Before the late 1980s, it could have been said that patient associations were generally much less concerned with the system of medicines regulation than consumer organisations or public health advocacy groups. However, the AIDS epidemic in the US and the large number of patients involved in litigation regarding the adverse effects of dependence on benzodiazepines in the UK have created much more politically active patient associations, such as the American AIDS Coalition To Unleash Power (ACT UP) and the British Tranquillizer Action Group (Epstein 1996; Walker 1993).

Consumer organisations, patient associations and public health advocacy organisations are all more active in the medical field in the US than their counterparts in Europe. For example, Public Citizen Health Research Group, based in Washington DC, is the largest public health advocacy group in the world and the organised political intervention of ACT UP is unrivalled by any other national patient association. Nevertheless, in the UK a considerable number of organised interests have developed in the last few decades. The two most substantial consumer organisations are the Consumers' Association (CA) and the National Consumer Council (NCC). The former houses and regularly publishes the *Drugs and Therapeutics Bulletin* – a critical guide to the safety and effectiveness of medicines for doctors and consumers. While the CA is funded independently via membership, the NCC is dependent on funding from central government. However, that dependence has not prevented the NCC from publishing several reports highly critical of medicines regulation in the UK and in Europe, especially with respect to lack of transparency and consumer representation in the decision-making process. The main public health advocacy group in the UK is Social Audit, under the direction of Charles Medawar, who has written many books and reports on the safety and value of pharmaceutical products for consumers over the last twenty-five years (e.g. Medawar 1984, 1992a).

In sharp contrast to the extensive environmentalist movement in Germany (Boehmer-Christiansen and Skea 1991), public health advocacy in the field of medicines has a fairly low profile, especially where prescription drugs are concerned. The main German consumer organisation is Stiftung Warentest, whose primary interest in medicines is with the safety and benefits of over-the-counter products. In general, German consumer organisations do not become involved with medicines regulation, except on a fairly informal basis.[3] Notably, in Germany since 1976 the legal provision of strict liability of manufacturers for damage caused by their drugs has been in place (Siehr 1986).[4]

Similarly, we found little *organised* consumer interest in pharmaceutical regulation in Sweden, where relatively inactive patient associations seem to be the primary form of collective representation. This may be because a more consensual political culture exists in Sweden than in the UK or Germany, as Kelman (1981) suggests, or it may be because citizens feel less need to campaign against potential drug risks because the state ensures that all Swedes are covered by liability insurance, supplemented by a no-fault compensation scheme – modestly funded by the Swedish drug industry. Thus, compared with Germany or Sweden, British patients and consumers have less recourse to compensation in the event of drug injury.

## The establishment of modern drug regulation

In broad terms, the initial stages of medicines regulation in Germany and the UK are quite similar. Before the 1960s, legislation in both countries provided only for governmental controls on drug quality, not the regulation of medicines' safety or efficacy. In that period, medicines regulation was crude, especially in Germany, while in the 1960s and 1970s both countries saw a flurry of regulatory activity concerning the safety and efficacy of medicines.

In the UK prior to the 1960s, drug quality was regulated by reference to the British Pharmacopoeia under the 1875 Sale of Food and Drugs Act. This was supplemented by the 1920 Dangerous Drugs Act, which made addictive drugs such as opium and cocaine prescription-only products, and the 1941 Pharmacy and Medicines Act, which prohibited the sale of drug products whose ingredients were not declared to the medical profession, and restricted the sale of some categories of medicines to pharmacists (Abraham 1995: 37–54). Similarly, in Germany the Imperial Order of 1872 on trade in drugs under the Kaiserreich attempted to regulate drug quality by restricting the sale of pharmaceuticals to recognised apothecaries. Well into the twentieth century, the German government limited drug regulation to manufacturing and distribution controls which were supported by the pharmacy and medical professions (Hancher and Reute 1984: 24–5).

One important difference between the two countries is that in 1943 the Nazi administration in Germany banned the production of all new drugs, except those specially sanctioned for the 'defence of the Reich'. As the ban was not lifted by the government of the Federal Republic of Germany (hereafter Germany) after World War II, in 1950 the pharmaceutical industry proposed a new drug law to reinstate licensing of drug manufacturers combined with a procedure for registering new drugs with a central government regulatory agency. For the industry, such regulation was preferable to a total ban on manufacturing. Remarkably, the German government rejected these proposals, arguing that the ban, albeit instituted by the Nazis, provided an important brake on the industry's tendency to market unnecessary and even dangerous drugs (Daemmrich 2000).

While German citizens continued to have access to new medicines produced and imported from overseas, the domestic ban was regarded by many as excessively authoritarian. For this reason, in 1959 the German Constitutional Court declared the ban to be unconstitutional. Consequently, German health authorities lost the only means at their disposal to control pharmaceutical manufacture and gain information on the type of drugs being marketed (Hancher and Reute 1984: 25). To fill this void, Parliament, with strong encouragement from the Constitutional Court, enacted the 1961 German Drug Law (*Arzneimittelein Gesetz*, or AMG).

The AMG 1961 created Germany's first modern drug regulatory authority, the Federal Health Ministry (Bundesgesundheitsamt, or BGA) and introduced compulsory registration of new medicines with the BGA. It established the licensing of manufacturers by the federal states (Länder) and required firms to report on pharmacological testing and adverse reactions to a new drug when registering it with the BGA. However, the BGA did not mandate specific tests. Nor did it have the power to refuse registration unless it could prove the new drug produced unacceptable effects in the post-marketing phase (Daemmrich 2000; Schmitt-Rau 1988). Unlike the modern regulation developed in Sweden and the UK, the control of biologicals, such as sera and vaccines, was the responsibility of an organisation (the Paul Erlich Institute) separate from the drug regulatory authority.

Later, in 1961, the thalidomide disaster illustrated the tremendous potential for harm that modern drugs possessed. The sedative was associated with approximately 10,000 birth defects worldwide. Soon after, the *Pharmaceutical Journal*, not renowned for radical criticism of the British regulatory system, carried an editorial stating:

> It is hard to imagine a more difficult choice than that which faces a manufacturer who has to decide whether or not to withdraw a profitable drug from the market on the basis of the evidence that, on the one hand, the drug may be dangerous to a small number of patients and, on the other, have valuable properties. So difficult must the choice be that it is questionable whether the manufacturer should be the one to make it.
>
> (Anon 1962a: 417–18)

Lord Cohen, chairman of the UK Health Ministry's Sub-committee of the Standing Medical Advisory Committees, was prompted to remark at a symposium in April 1962 that in the previous year more than half the drugs which had been issued had not been correctly clinically tested, and that there was ample evidence of manufacturers supplying biased and unreliable information to physicians (Anon 1962b; Anon 1962d). Later that year his committee advised the British government that there should be an advisory body to review the evidence and offer advice on the toxicity of new drugs, but that it was 'neither desirable nor practicable' to establish a central drug testing authority (ABPI 1963; Anon 1962c).

In response, the British government set up a system of pre-market clearance for new drugs, on the basis of safety and efficacy assessments made by experts on a new advisory body known as the Committee on Safety of Drugs (CSD), while the industry remained in control of drug testing operations. Significantly, the CSD arrangement was voluntary and did not have the force of law. The Health Minister appointed Sir Derrick Dunlop as chairman of the CSD and pronounced that its membership were of such eminence that it was unthinkable that they would submit to any influence but the force of scientific considerations (Anon 1963a). However that may be, five of the twelve members of the CSD had backgrounds in the pharmaceutical industry, and members of the committee were permitted to hold consultancies with, and shares in, drug companies without disclosing them to the public (Anon 1963b). Dunlop himself was later to move to a senior position in the industry (Gould 1972). Furthermore, some members evidently assumed the best about industrial drug testing. For example, in 1962 Professor Wilson held the conviction that:

if a drug is shown to be harmful to animals, its use in Man is not contemplated ... and every reputable pharmaceutical firm and clinical investigator ensures to the best of current knowledge that all the appropriate investigations have been done before the drug is given to Man.

(Wilson 1962: 196)

Within its terms of reference the CSD was to invite reports on toxicity tests from the manufacturer, consider whether the drug should be put to clinical trial, obtain reports of such trials, and take into account the safety, efficacy and adverse effects of the drug (Anon 1963b). It began operations on 1 January 1964, and the ABPI undertook not to market or submit to clinical trial any new drug against the advice of the Committee (Anon 1963c). Two months beforehand, the CSD had pledged that information submitted to it by manufacturers about new drugs would be treated as confidential to the Committee, ostensibly to ensure that the development of new drugs of therapeutic value was not hindered (Anon 1963d).

As Cahal, the CSD's Medical Assessor, explained, the Committee was dependent on the industry's co-operation: 'One is often asked how the Committee manages to comply with its terms of reference with so small staff. The answer is "decentralisation", which means, since there is nowhere else to which we can decentralise, decentralisation to industry' (US Congress 1970: 37).

Such extensive contact with industry, however, was not without impact on the way the CSD conducted itself, as Wade, a former member, later explained:

> Looking back I see only one major error in our performance. We were so aware of the enormous cooperation that we received from the drug industry that the main Committee made every effort it could to see that submissions from firms were handled as rapidly as possible – as a result ... the Adverse Reactions subcommittee and ... the work of that subcommittee suffered.
>
> (Wade 1983: 3)

Regulatory review was indeed rapid, averaging three months for NASs and one month for novel reformulations (Anon 1966). This was a deliberate policy, as is clear from the CSD's annual report for 1966: 'it is fully recognised that a Committee such as this might exercise a detrimental effect on pharmaceutical research progress by unduly delaying the introduction of a possibly valuable drug or even by preventing its use altogether' (Anon 1967: 59–60).

In 1965 and 1966 the CSD refused to approve only about 2 per cent of new drug applications, but accepted over 75 per cent. Even in 1970, the CSD's most established and last full year of operation, the Committee refused less than 6 per cent of applications.

Meanwhile, in Germany, where thalidomide was marketed as Contergan, widespread use of the sedative, available without prescription, led to approximately 4,000 cases of phocomelia among German children born between 1959 and 1962.[5] In response, the AMG 1961 was strengthened in 1964 by introducing the requirement that reports supplied on drug registration had to be supported by documentary evidence. Manufacturers also had to give written assurances that products had been tested in accordance with the scientific standards of the appropriate professional organisations, such as the German Society for Internal Medicine and the German Pharmacological Society (Daemmrich 2000). Furthermore, the 1964 law required new medicines to be available on prescription only for a minimum of three years, and gave the BGA powers to forbid marketing if the data supplied on registration was incomplete or if the drug seemed likely to be hazardous or ineffective (Daemmrich 2000; Hancher and Reute 1984: 26–7).

Appreciating that the CSD could be only an interim measure, the UK Labour government passed the Medicines Act in 1968, which legally required drug manufacturers to obtain approval from the government for clinical trials with patients and the marketing of new drug products. Approval of the former was defined by a clinical trial certificate, and of the latter by a product licence. This Act formed the basis for the regulatory control of pharmaceuticals in the UK up to 1995 (when many aspects of it were superseded by EU legislation – see Chapter 4). To obtain a product licence (also known as marketing authorisation) under the Act, manufacturers needed to submit adequate scientific evidence of safety and efficacy to the government's Licensing Authority, then known as the Medicines Division of the Department of Health. A product licence had to be accompanied by a 'data sheet', which outlined the indications, contraindications, adverse effects and other information about the drug. Under the 1968 Medicines Act, it became an offence for a manufacturer to advertise a drug product to doctors without supplying the data sheet. In this respect, the Act also significantly extended regulation of labelling and advertising in the pharmaceutical sector (Anon 1968).

Under the 1968 Medicines Act a number of expert advisory bodies were created to assist the Licensing Authority in medicines regulation, most notably the Medicines Commission and the highly influential Committee on Safety of Medicines (CSM) – in effect, the successor of the CSD. The members of both these advisory bodies are appointed by the Health Minister. Typically, the membership of the Medicines Commission is drawn from academic medical and veterinary sciences, toxicology, clinical practice, medical law, ethics and the pharmaceutical industry, whereas the membership of the CSM consists solely of scientists. The Medicines Commission advises the Minister on the appointment of expert scientific committees, such as the CSM, and acts as an appellate body for pharmaceutical companies who feel aggrieved by a decision to refuse or revoke a product licence (Cmnd 3395 1967; Medicines Act 1968). However, before making such a decision, the Licensing Authority is required to consult with the appropriate expert scientific committee, such as the CSM. It is also required to seek the opinion of the CSM before approving a new drug for marketing.

The new regulations were not confined to product licensing. Manufacturers were also required to submit a full application in order to obtain a licence to conduct new clinical trials. Such applications were to meet the regulators' guidelines on supporting data concerning the quality and toxicity of the trial drug. The CSM also established a system for monitoring the safety of medicines after they have reached the market, by encouraging doctors to report suspected adverse drug reactions (ADRs) as they occurred in clinical practice. This post-marketing surveillance of voluntary spontaneous reporting became known as the 'yellow card system', because doctors completed yellow forms when making the reports. In addition, under the Medicines Act there is a legal requirement for pharmaceutical companies to report suspected ADRs to their products to the Licensing Authority. The pharmacovigilance data generated by these various aspects of post-marketing surveillance became integrated into the regulatory activity of the Medicines Division.

As Hancher and Reute (1984) note, the 1964 drug law in Germany marked a decisive shift *towards* a product licensing system, like that established by the UK Medicines Act, although the criteria for assessing safety and efficacy were not yet established by the BGA. The voluntary guidelines on safety and efficacy testing drawn up by the medical profession in 1964 were replaced by administrative guidelines in 1971, which were legally binding on the BGA and instructed the regulatory authority not to permit approval unless clinical trials met them. However, these guidelines were not legally binding on manufacturers and applied only to new drugs, but not generic or established products. To remedy these defects, and to bring German legislation into line with an EU directive regarding the pre-market review of drug safety and efficacy by Member States, the 1976 German Drug Law (AMG 1976) was introduced (Schmitt-Rau 1988).

The AMG 1976 marked a substantial change to a much more interventionist style of regulation compared with the market-orientated approach of AMG 1961. It introduced criteria of safety, efficacy and quality, and established post-marketing monitoring of approved drugs. Like the UK Medicines Act of 1968, the AMG 1976 was comprehensive in its coverage of matters relating to manufacture and marketing. For example, the BGA mandated drug testing regimes and required product licence applications to include basic pre-clinical and clinical data on a new drug's composition, toxicity, clinical pharmacology and efficacy. In some ways, it went further by including detailed requirements on ADR reporting, the training of sales representatives and a system of compensation for patients suffering drug injury based on absolute liability (Hancher and Reute 1984). Under the AMG 1976, the BGA formed 'approval commissions', which were like the expert scientific advisory committee created in the UK about ten years before, but with less influence. Unlike the UK Medicines Act, which envisaged a central role for the CSM in the British regulatory system, the recommendations of the German approval commissions could be bypassed by the BGA so long as a justification was provided to the manufacturer (Daemmrich 2000).

In Sweden, medicines regulation advanced much earlier than in Germany or the UK. In fact, the Nordic countries were among the first to introduce drug regulation relating to safety and efficacy. Sweden first developed such controls over approval and marketing in 1934, while Norwegian legislation dates from 1928 (Lee and Herzstein 1986). As Dukes (1985) notes, this early adoption of efficacy criteria challenges the claim that the need for proof of efficacy did not (and could not) occur for regulatory purposes until the growth of clinical pharmacology in the 1960s and 1970s.

Since 1935, Swedish drug laws have required manufacturers to demonstrate the safety and efficacy of their products prior to approval by the national drug regulatory authority, then known as the Department of Drugs (the SLA) within the National Board of Health and Welfare (NBHW). It is probably for this reason that the number of medicinal products in Sweden has been considerably lower than in Germany or the UK. In practice, the SLA was assisted with approval decisions by a scientific advisory board for drug registration. The advisory board was replaced in the 1960s by the Board of Drugs (BOD) on whom was conferred the responsibility of arriving at the final decisions on drug approvals, although the Board always included three representatives of the SLA *ex officio*. While the BOD made the final decision, the SLA continued to conduct the primary analysis of the new drug applications, supplying the Board with a summary evaluation of the submitted data and a recommendation of acceptance or rejection of the application (Liljestrand 1979). In order to gain final approval, companies had to submit a 'data sheet', known as a FASS sheet, summarising the characteristics of the product. At this time, the Board also compiled a list of about 2,500 approved drugs based on safety, efficacy, accuracy of promotion and reasonable pricing (Dukes 1985). Indeed, in the 1990s the number of medicinal products on the Swedish market remained as low as 3,000, compared with about 8,000 in the UK and 50,000 in Germany – by far the largest European market and worth about US$17 billion (Anon 1990i: 6; Anon 1998s; Apoteksbolaget 1994; Hildebrandt 1995b: 909).

From the mid-1960s to 1981, the BOD had been more powerful than its British counterpart, the CSM. However, the roles of the BOD and the SLA were changed in 1981, when attempts were made to make the Department more autonomous from the NBHW, following the American style of semi-independent regulatory agencies. However, the Swedish government prevented such attempts and moved to *constrain* the Department's autonomy by making the Director General of the SLA also the chairman of the BOD. Simultaneously, the BOD became solely advisory, losing its power of final decision-making to the Director General of the SLA. Thus, since 1981, the BOD has become, in effect, an advisory committee like the CSM, but with less autonomy or influence because it is now chaired by the Director General of the regulatory authority, who has final decision-making power.

Unlike Germany and the UK, Sweden already had pre-market safety and efficacy regulations in place before thalidomide, though this did not prevent the drug receiving marketing authorisation there as Meurosedyn. This highlighted the importance of post-market monitoring of drug safety as well as pre-market controls. Thus, in 1965 the Swedish Department of Drugs established its Adverse Drug Reaction Committee (ADRC), which collected and reviewed doctors' voluntary reporting of suspected adverse reactions to drugs on the market. A tradition was established that doctors reported suspected ADRs directly to the regulatory authorities rather than to companies. By all accounts, this system has been more successful than its British or German counterparts, partly because Swedish doctors have been more conscientious about filing such reports with the ADRC and partly because there are fewer medicines to track (Bottiger 1988). As Liljestrand (1979) put it:

> From an international point of view our [the Swedish] national system for spontaneous monitoring of adverse reactions has been fairly successful. A cooperative and homogeneous body of physicians and a reasonably small number of drugs on the market facilitating observations on cause–effect relationships have been of great help.
>
> (Liljestrand 1979: 36)

It has also been easier for Swedish regulators to monitor the sales of drugs than in many other European countries, because retail sale of all medicines, except natural products, has been through a single company, Apoteksbolaget. It was also established in the early 1960s in response to thalidomide, and is jointly owned by the state and its own pension fund (Apoteksbolaget 1994). This state pharmacy company has set up 'active drug committees' in all major hospitals, and by 1990 was also covering about half of outpatient care in Sweden, providing information and feedback on prescribing and consumption patterns to all those involved in the handling of pharmaceuticals (Anon 1990b: 3).

## 'Independence' and 'conflict of interest'

Lord Cohen's committee had recommended that the British CSD should be 'entirely independent of industry', but as we noted, members of the CSD were permitted to, and did, retain consultancies with pharmaceutical companies (Department of Health 1971: 8). In 1970, however, the Department of Health invited the ABPI to consider a change of policy whereby persons holding consultancies in the industry would not be appointed to the CSD or its subcommittees. The ABPI, who hoped that the new regulatory system would mimic the CSD's informal and flexible approach to industry, refused to support such a change, and it was never made (ABPI 1971). Indeed, all the major elements of regulatory organisations in the UK concerned with drug safety and efficacy have

exhibited a close relationship with the pharmaceutical industry via
direct representation, consultancies or prior and/or subsequent
employment (Anon 1991b; Collier 1985; Delamothe 1989). For
example, John Griffin, who was medical director of a pharmaceutical company before joining the Department of Health's
Medicines Division in 1971, the CSM's Secretariat, resigned from
his position as Head of the Medicines Division in 1984 in order to
take up the Directorship of the ABPI. On joining the ABPI, he
revealed that the extent of exchange of personnel between industry
and the Medicines Division went well beyond his own case:

> All my deputies [at the Medicines Division], principal medical
> officers, have been in industry. All the superintendent pharma-
> cists that I had working for me, all came from industry. It is
> equally clear that within the last 12 months I am not the only
> member of the medical staff of the division to move back into
> industry.
>
> (ABPI 1984: 3)

Given the longevity of Griffin's important position at the
Medicines Division, his views about the extent of such exchange
are significant. This industry–regulator 'revolving door' was not
without cause or consequence. As Griffin put it:

> It is abundantly clear to me that the Medicines Division could
> not function if it did not recruit the expertise that it requires
> from the industry. I have always opposed the development of
> any attitude which I could only classify as adversarial, and I have
> resisted any attempts by either the industry, the permanent staff
> of the Medicines Division, or the committees to adopt an adver-
> sarial role. The role of the regulators is in fact to achieve the
> release on to the market of those products which have had peer
> review which has shown them as satisfactory for the indications
> for which they were going to be marketed.
>
> (ABPI 1984: 3)

Quantitative data regarding the industrial interests of the expert
scientific advisors to the British drug regulatory authorities
remained confidential to Ministers until the late 1980s. When
made publicly available, these data showed that, in 1989, only a
fifth of the expert advisers on the CSM or the Medicines

Commission had neither personal nor non-personal financial
interests in the industry. In 1996 the figure remained as low as a
quarter (Table 3.1). Of the twenty-three members of the CSM
with financial interests in 1996, three had interests in at least
twenty companies, seven had interests in at least ten companies,
and twenty members had interests in at least five companies
(MCA 1997: 81–90).

The situation in Germany and Sweden is similar to that in the
UK regarding conflicts of interest. Members of the Swedish BOD
and the German Approval Commissions have been permitted to
retain personal and non-personal financial interests in the pharmaceutical industry. However, there exists some scepticism about
how rigorously declarations of conflicts of interests have been
applied to German Approval Commissions, if at all (Anon
1992e). One contrast with the UK is that, even during the 1990s,
Swedish and German expert advisors were not required to publish
non-personal interests, such as industry funding for their
academic research. On the other hand, on occasions the Swedish
regulatory authorities are known to have rejected proposed
members of the BOD because their links with industry were
considered to be too great. Another difference between the UK, on
the one hand, and Germany and Sweden, on the other, is that there
is very little public debate about conflicts of interest in medicines
regulation in the latter two countries. This may be a reflection of

*Table 3.1*   Industrial interests of expert scientific advisers on
medicines regulation in 1989 and 1996

|  | *Personal interests*[a] | *Non-personal interests*[b] | *Neither* |
|---|---|---|---|
| Med Commission (n = 24 [19][c]) | 17 [11] | 7 [7] | 5 [6] |
| CSM (n = 21 [29] | 14 [18] | 15 [22] | 4 [6] |
| Total (n = 45 [48]) | 31 [29] | 22 [29] | 9 [12] |

*Source:*   Delamothe 1989: 476; MCA 1997: 78–90

*Notes:*
[a] defined as consultancies, fee-paid work and shareholding
[b] defined as payments that benefit department for which member is responsible
but are not received by member personally
[c] [ ] = figures for 1996

the comparatively low level of organised consumer interest and public health advocacy within Germany and Sweden.

## Neo-liberal politics and the minimal regulatory state

During the 1970s, the ABPI maintained its strategic influence over the UK Licensing Authority and its advisory committees on drug safety through close consultation about regulations on data requirements for clinical trial certificates (CTCs) and product licences (ABPI 1972). Nevertheless, the regulatory authorities did demand increasingly detailed and complex pre-clinical data before granting CTCs. In 1977, just over one-third of CTC applications were granted without requesting further information, compared with 74 per cent in 1971 (CSD 1972: 12; CSM 1978: 28). Furthermore, it was claimed that the average time before clinical testing in the UK was four times that required in several other major Western countries (Cromie 1980). Consequently, the number of CTCs issued fell from 170 in 1972 to 87 in 1980, and, according to industry representatives, companies shifted investment in clinical trials to locations outside the UK (ABPI 1977a; Griffin and Diggle 1981: 461).

Neither these controls nor the yellow card monitoring system managed to prevent several thousand patients in Britain suffering severe adverse effects after taking ICI's beta-blocking drug, practolol (Eraldin), in the mid-1970s (Lesser 1977). At the time, practolol was the biggest drug disaster recorded in the UK, provoking a search for more effective forms of regulating drug safety (ABPI 1977b; Anon 1976; Anon 1978). In 1975, the Committee on the Review of Medicines (CRM) was established to comply with the EU directive requiring all medicines to be assessed according to modern licensing standards by 1990. The task involved reviewing some 36,000 medicinal products, including over 4,000 prescription drugs, which had been permitted to stay on the market when the 1968 Medicines Act came into force, without any examination of whether they were safe or effective by the UK regulatory authorities (Anon 1977; Binns 1980).

The industry was reluctant to assist a body which threatened to restrict or revoke existing licences. Moreover, to accelerate the review process, the Minister of Health decided that consultation procedures with industry should be bypassed for products which the CRM thought to present a particular hazard to public health. As a result, the industry and regulatory authorities in the UK drifted into an 'adversarial attitude' (Hurley 1983: 3). For example, the CRM was challenged in the courts by the industry about some recommendations to revoke product licences (Hancher 1989). While industrial interests continued to be influential, it was not until 1979, when the Conservatives came to power under Margaret Thatcher, that their concerns were received with an enthusiastic ear from government.

The Conservatives were elected with a positive commitment to reduce state intervention in the economy, and medicines regulation was no exception. From March 1981, the Thatcher Government introduced a clinical trial exemption scheme in which a manufacturer needed only to submit a summary of the data relevant for a CTC to the Department of Health's Medicines Division, who then had five weeks to object to the proposed trials (ABPI 1981; DHSS 1981). If the regulators made no objections, then the trials could proceed. The scheme was much welcomed by industry (Smart 1981). Senior representatives of the Medicines Division stated that the scheme had become necessary 'because early developmental work on new drugs was going abroad to the detriment of British industry' (Griffin and Long 1981: 477). Thus, the UK regulatory authority had adopted both the industry's interpretation of the effects of the earlier more stringent CTC requirements and its suggestions for change, even though research has shown retrospectively that, in the period 1972 to 1983, on average, NASs came to the UK market faster than in France, Germany, Italy, Sweden or the US (Andersson 1992: 62). Moreover, during the 1970s pharmaceutical regulation grew more slowly than in most other sectors in the UK, such as occupational health and safety, environmental pollution, consumer protection and town and country planning (Peacock 1984: 46).

During the 1980s, the ABPI complained that the Medicines Division was 'inefficient' and too conservative about approving drugs. In particular, the industry continued to badger the British government and regulatory authorities to organise medicines control according to the industry's desire for faster drug approvals. The Thatcher Government, which was already planning a programme of 'reform' of the civil service, responded sympathetically by turning its neo-liberal agenda to medicines regulation (Anon 1988b). In 1987, it instigated a review of the Medicines Division, asking two consultants, Dr John Evans and Peter Cunliffe, to conduct it. Though few realised it at the time, this development marked the beginning of a significant shift towards a 'lighter touch' regulatory philosophy in the UK, which was to outlast the century and eventually influence other European countries.

In response, the ABPI submitted proposals to what became known as the Cunliffe/Evans Inquiry. The industry suggested that it would be willing to pay the costs of funding drug approvals if this were to result in a 'more efficient service' (Anon 1988a: 3). The ABPI also called for greater dialogue and informal consultation between companies and regulators in the Licensing Authority and the CSM about the assessment of new drug applications (Anon 1987a). Many of these sentiments were shared by Professor William Asscher, then chairman of the CSM, who commented that the CSM was already taking steps to improve its speed and accuracy in regulatory advice together with its level of communication with pharmaceutical companies. He hoped that the Cunliffe/Evans Inquiry would suggest ways in which the Medicines Division could do the same (Anon 1987b).

But there was an alternative account of the situation at the Medicines Division, rarely heard at that time, and apparently not substantially on the Cunliffe/Evans agenda. In fact, the British drug regulatory authority had been starved of resources during the Thatcher Government. In the ten years to 1986, licence applications of all types had increased by 87 per cent, while staff levels in the Medicines Division grew by only 9 per cent. In the late 1980s, the American drug regulatory agency had six times as many staff handling drug applications as the UK Licensing Authority (Anon 1989i: 3). This suggests that the Medicines Division may not have been structurally inefficient, but merely under-resourced by the state. Further evidence, which casts doubt on the validity of the claim that the Medicines Division was inefficient, is that from 1961 to 1985 more NASs were first marketed in the UK than in Austria, the Benelux countries, the Eastern bloc, Italy, Scandinavia, Spain, Switzerland or the US, and in 1988 the UK was found to have the fastest approval times for new drugs in the EU (Andersson 1992: 68; Anon 1988f).

During the 1970s and 1980s, about 60 per cent of the annual running costs of the Medicines Division were recouped from the pharmaceutical industry through licence fees, while 40 per cent of funding came from the Treasury via taxation. Cunliffe and Evans accepted the industry's proposal that, in order to make medicines control more 'efficient', the entire cost of running the regulatory authority (an estimated £12 million in 1988) should be dependent on fees paid by pharmaceutical companies for licensing. Moreover, they recommended that a Budget Committee, composed of representatives of the industry, the Department of Health and the Treasury, should meet twice a year to monitor the cost and efficiency of the regulatory authority. A new director post for the regulatory agency, employed on a contract basis, was to be held to account for the performance of the regulatory authority by the Budget Committee and the Department of Health, while within the authority new 'businesses' with 'team leaders' were also to be responsible for their staff's performance. The Cunliffe/Evans report also echoed the industry's view that communication between companies and regulators had become too formal since the 1968 Medicines Act and recommended that more informal communication should be encouraged (Anon 1988a).

In 1989, the UK government accepted the main recommendations made by Cunliffe and Evans. A new industry-funded regulatory authority, known as the Medicines Control Agency (MCA), with its own director and budgetary consultative group, was created in place of the Medicines Division (Anon 1989a). The new director of the MCA, Dr Keith Jones, came from industry, having spent the previous ten years at Merck, Sharp and Dohme and some years before that at Beecham and Fison (Anon 1989e). On arrival, he set about establishing 'business units' within the MCA and announced that the agency aimed to reduce the net processing times for new drugs by 24 per cent within a year (Anon 1989i: 2).

There were five functional 'business units': New Drugs Licensing; Abridged Licensing; Pharmacovigilance; Inspection and Enforcement; and Executive Support. The first four of these conducted scientific work to inform regulation of drug safety, efficacy and quality, while the fifth provided organisational infrastructure, including policy co-ordination. Notably, the Pharmacovigilance business unit developed the Adverse Drug Reactions On-line Information Tracking Unit (ADROIT) – the MCA's computerised system of collating spontaneous post-market reports of suspected ADRs – and in collaboration with the CSM electronic reporting of suspected ADRs was permitted in the late 1990s (Anon 1998c; MCA 1993a: 71–84).

After 1994, a few minor organisational changes were made: New Drugs Licensing and Abridged Licensing merged into a single business unit called Licensing; and the Pharmacovigilance business unit changed its name to 'Post-Licensing', probably to reflect the fact that its work involved the control of medicines promotion and labelling as well as post-market surveillance of drug safety (MCA 1996: 18–19).[6] Relations with the CSM remained essentially unchanged – the MCA continued to deal with about 90 per cent of applications without referral to the committee, while always seeking its advice regarding new drug applications and very rarely rejecting that advice (MCA 1993a: 29).[7] However, this does not imply that the CSM was unaffected by the changing regulatory culture. The committee established new procedures to accelerate its own role in the drug review process. In 1987, the CSM advised the granting of a licence on first consideration (without resubmission) for 35 per cent of new drug applications – a figure which had risen to 56 per cent by 1995 (CSM 1996; Rawlins and Jefferys 1993).

Negotiations over the licensing fees for new drugs revealed the 'exchange' underpinning the new arrangements. For example, industry objected to paying a licensing fee as large as £50,000 for a new drug application without any assurance that their products would pass more quickly through the regulatory system – a sum of £40,000 was finally agreed (Anon 1989f). Despite the fact that some Labour MPs expressed concern that the MCA might not be truly independent because it was being wholly financed by the pharmaceutical industry, the Under-Secretary of State for Health, Roger Freeman, told Parliament that reducing the time taken by the MCA to process licence applications was a good investment for the industry (Anon 1989g).

At the MCA's first annual symposium in November 1990, Kenneth Clarke, the Secretary of State for Health, welcomed the introduction of the new agency because, he suggested, the Medicines Division had lacked success in providing an effective and efficient service to the industry. He also noted that the organisational changes made at the MCA were much in line with the Thatcher Government's 'reform programme' for the civil service, in which the executive functions of government should be carried out by 'executive agencies' within departments, led by chief executives with responsibility for day-to-day operations (Anon 1990h: 2). However, in its first year, the MCA showed an operating loss of £2.9 million (Anon 1990j). To cope with this, the MCA's budgetary consultative group, consisting of senior officials from the Department of Health, the MCA and industry, decided that the licensing fees paid by industry needed to increase by 70 per cent in 1990. For example, the fee for processing a new drug application increased from £40,000 to £68,000 (Anon 1989n: 1). In its second year, the agency was mounting debts approaching £3.8 million, so it raised licensing fees even more from December 1990: the fee for processing a new drug application rose by 90 per cent, from £68,000 to £130,000 (Anon 1990f; 1991a). In general, manufacturers continued to bear these escalating costs because they still represented a small proportion of overall R and D costs, though small manufacturers, such as the Natural Medicines Group and the British Herbal Medicines Association, had difficulties and even challenged the fee increases in court – unsuccessfully (Anon 1990c).

The strategy of increasing fees from industry eventually paid dividends. In July 1991, the MCA announced that it had achieved a surplus of about £1.8 million and had become financially self-supporting, with an income of about £13.4 million derived from fees paid by the pharmaceutical industry (Anon 1991g). The following year, the agency recorded even greater surpluses as its income from industry fees rose to about £19.6 million (Anon 1992d). The MCA also seems to have succeeded in increasing its contact and consultation with industry via regulatory staff at individual companies and briefing meetings with the ABPI. Contrary to the situation in the late 1980s, we found that industry generally perceived the MCA as being very accessible for consultation and advice in the late 1990s. Such 'progress' did not go unnoticed by the British government, which awarded the MCA with 'executive agency' status. Stephen Dorrell, the Under-Secretary for Health, noted that the MCA had become self-sufficient through fees paid by industry, thus saving the taxpayer £7 million per year. The 'executive agency' status meant that Keith Jones, as chief executive, had greater budgetary and management flexibility as he became free from the requirement to report to senior civil servants, though he remained accountable to Ministers (Anon 1991f; MCA 1991a).

As an 'executive agency', the MCA's objectives and functions became defined, in effect, by a contract between the agency, the Department of Health and the Health Ministers (MCA 1991a;

MCA 1993a: 69). A concise formulation of the agency's objectives, which states its 'dual responsibilities' to both patients and industry, is provided in the following passage from a promotional brochure:

> Overall, the agency aims to provide an efficient, cost-effective service that protects the users of medicines while not impeding the effectiveness of the pharmaceutical industry. Indeed, the MCA positively encourages the development of new medicines which are in the interests of public health.
>
> (MCA 1991b: 1)

At this time, Health Ministers also appointed a board of experts, drawn from various quarters including industry and the Department of Health, to advise them on the scope of the MCA's targets and its performance (Anon 1991f). With such sharply rising licensing fees, the MCA was keen to show that progress had been made to accelerate the drug approval process, and that the industry was getting 'value for money' (Anon 1990e: 2). In 1988, the average *gross* time taken to approve a new drug was 21 months, with the longest being 54 months, including time taken for advice from the CSM, informal discussions between manufacturers and regulators and for manufacturers to reply to letters from the regulators about the application. However, more pertinent to the MCA's efforts to accelerate drug approvals were the *net in-house* assessment times, which averaged 154 working days (about 31 weeks) for new drugs in 1989 (Anon 1989i). Net assessment times for new drugs were reduced by 40 per cent to 93 working days in 1990, 75 in 1991, 67 in 1993, and had dropped to just 44 by 1998. The number of licences granted for new drugs also increased, from 57 in 1989 to 77 in 1990, and remained as high as 79 in 1993 (Anon 1990e; Anon 1991d; Anon 1991m; Anon 1993l; Anon 1998r; MCA 1995; MCA 1996: 12–14).

The British government's strong approval for the new MCA approach to medicines regulation was signalled by the salary rewards to the agency's staff, most notably the chief executive, who received a bonus in 1992 bringing his salary up to over £78,000, up by 14 per cent on the previous year (Anon 1992d). Despite the elevated fees, pharmaceutical companies also seemed to be impressed: during the 1990s, about 40 per cent of applications to market drugs via the optional European regulatory procedures chose the MCA, rather than any other EU regulatory agency, as the rapporteur to conduct the assessment (Anon 1993h: 3). As the chief executive of the MCA was quick to note, this positioned the UK strongly in the bid for the siting of a new European drug regulatory agency planned for 1995 (Anon 1990g). This met with further approval from the British government. At the MCA's third annual symposium, the Parliamentary Secretary for Health made it clear that he wanted the new European agency in the UK, citing the MCA's quick approval times and leading position in European licensing work as strong points in the UK bid (Anon 1992g).

Others were not so enthusiastic. Doubts were expressed privately by other regulators in the EU about how any regulatory agency can remain independent of the pharmaceutical industry and act as a representative of the public interest while it is completely dependent on the industry's fees for its funding (Brown 1990). These reservations were not aimed solely at the MCA but also at events in Sweden, which seemed to follow the British trend. In Sweden, medicines regulation was already almost entirely funded by licensing fees from industry (Anon 1988e). However, in 1988, the Swedish Audit Office proposed that drug regulatory activity at the Department of Drugs should be removed from the National Board of Health and Welfare and given to a separate regulatory agency.

The proposals were made in the light of complaints from the industry that drug approval times were too long. The Audit Office highlighted the lengthy drug review process as 'a fundamental problem' with the Department of Drugs, and argued that a separate drug regulatory agency would be better placed to co-ordinate all aspects of the drug review process, including increases in recruitment and licensing fees, leading to greater 'efficiency'. The Swedish pharmaceutical industry association welcomed the proposals, commenting that the increased fees proposed by the Audit Office would be acceptable to the industry if they resulted in faster approval times (Anon 1988c). Research has shown that between 1972 and 1983 NASs came to the market in Sweden more slowly, on average, than in France, Germany, Italy, the UK or the US (Andersson 1992: 62, 68).

In the debate about the future of Swedish medicines regulation which followed the Audit Office report, the Department of Drugs argued that it was not a matter of making an inefficient organisation more efficient, but rather of providing the opportunity for an already effective organisation to cope with the size of its task by recruiting more staff. The implication – but only an implication – was that faster approval times did not necessarily equate with efficiency or progress in drug regulation. The Department of Drugs also responded defensively on the industry's terms of productivity by pointing to the fact that the gross mean of processing times for all types of applications had fallen from 18 to 15 months between 1987 and 1989 (Anon 1989b; Anon 1989m). However, the gross approval times for *new drug* applications grew from 27 to 33 months between 1988 and 1989 (Anon 1989m).

In 1990, the Swedish regulatory authority was established as an independent unit, the Medical Products Agency (MPA), with Professor Kjell Strandberg as Director General. Unlike the British MCA, there was no reference to 'business units', but some internal changes to the regulatory agency included a special task force, set up to reduce the backlog of applications and to provide more regular meetings about applications and internal peer review sessions on drug reviews, prior to committee meetings on whether or not to recommend approval. The MPA's fee structure put much more emphasis on 'annual fees' than the MCA. The licensing fee for regulatory review of a new drug application by the MPA in 1990 was set at SKr68,900 (US$11,500), but if the drug was approved, then thereafter the firm was required to pay an annual fee of about SKr57,500 (US$9,500) to subsidise the agency's post-marketing surveillance of the new product. Hence, in total, the fee for having a new drug approved by the MPA in 1990 was about US$20,000 in the first year, substantially less than the fee charged by the MCA (Anon 1990a).

By 1993, the MPA had reduced the mean gross approval times for new drug applications from 33 months in 1989 to 13 months (Anon 1994d). In 1994, the agency managed to review half of its new drug applications within 210 days, though the mean gross time for all products was 12 months (Anon 1995f). Evidently, the acceleration of drug approval times was debated publicly in response to industry concerns, and the MPA concentrated its efforts and resources on trying to reduce them, with considerable success. However, a rather different approach was taken towards rejections of new drug applications. Previously, product application rejections were published by the Swedish regulatory authorities (Anon 1990d). In response to industry requests, in 1993 the MPA agreed not to publish the fact that any application had been rejected. Moreover, the agency *extended* the response period for a company whose product licence application faced rejection from 6 weeks to 3 months (Anon 1993a).

The industry's concerns about drug approval times achieved a new prominence when specific time frames were recommended in Sweden's Medicinal Product Act, which together with the Medicinal Products Ordinance came into force on 1 July 1993. This legislation defined the framework for the marketing of medicines in Sweden up to 1995 (when many aspects were superseded by EU legislation – see Chapter 4). It did not introduce fundamental changes to Swedish drug regulation, but did recommend that MPA evaluation of licensing applications should be completed within specified times. While not mandatory, the agency is expected to treat these time frames as internal institutional goals. For example, it was recommended that assessments of new drug applications should be completed within 210 days.

During the 1990s, the MPA has grown to employ about 200 staff (MPA 1996a). In 1993, it was reorganised into thirteen production units, also known as 'results units', two of which were devoted to evaluating licensing applications while others concentrated on areas such as pharmacovigilance, toxicology research, clinical trials and inspection. According to the agency, its working style is 'project orientated and target driven', encouraging consultation with industry: 'Dialogue and openness, within our organisation and with our clients, require flexible exchange of information. Accordingly, we are creating an organisation based on internal and external networks and project groups adapted to needs and the special work situations' (MPA 1996b: 3).

According to some industry sources, the 1990s have seen frequent communication between MPA assessors and applicant firms during the drug review process.

As well as entering into dialogue with industry, the MPA also produces publications encouraging rational prescribing practices and other materials for health professionals on drug information and recommended treatments. Significantly, the MPA advises doctors on the relative benefits of different treatments, which goes further than the kind of information published by the British CSM or MCA but is not dissimilar from the approach of the UK Consumers' Association's *Drugs and Therapeutics Bulletin*. Indeed, one official at the MCA criticised the MPA's publications for being 'a sort of scientific analysis', rather than being 'regulatory information' that is 'straight factual stuff'.[8]

The 1993 Act introduced an authorisation system regarding clinical trials to replace the previous notification system. In practice, this meant little change because an approval system was already functional. Also, under the Act, a document called the 'summary of product characteristics', approved by the MPA, became the official label for new drugs on which the 'old' FASS sheet published by the LIF had to be based. The legislation made no changes to relations between the MPA and the BOD. Final decisions continued to rest with the Director General of the MPA, who remained chair of the BOD. Like the CSM, the BOD is not involved in every application, but reviews normally give advice on all new drug applications. Unlike the CSM, the members of the BOD are appointed by the MPA rather than by Ministers. It is rare for the MPA and the BOD to reach conflicting decisions. As one MPA scientist put it:

> There has always been a procedure to come to a compromise
> ... If there are differences of opinion within the agency, the
> chairman and the Board, we've always managed to come up
> to a unified solution. So it's very seldom that there's been any
> conflict.[9]

According to the secretary of the BOD, on no occasion has the Director General of the MPA made a decision contrary to the wishes of the Board. As the secretary explained, such a situation could have severe consequences because it would undermine the authority of the BOD:

> I can say that it would be very odd if the Director General is
> sitting in one meeting and taking one decision, but in the
> other room, at a later moment, he's taking another decision
> against the Board. It would be very peculiar indeed, but there
> is no such example. Of course, then the result would be that
> the Board of Drugs, the members, sitting there should say, if
> you do that, then we will finish here, because then there is no
> point in our coming here and making our decisions.[10]

Companies' rights against regulatory decisions remained much more limited than in the UK. There can be no appeal against decisions taken by the Director General of the MPA, MPA evaluations or advisory recommendations made by the BOD, but companies may withdraw an application which is going to be rejected. They also have the option of appealing against a negative decision by taking their case to the Administrative Court in Stockholm. However, in practice, few companies seek to resolve disputes through the courts. Three factors seem to account for this: the litigation process is slow; the courts nearly always support the MPA; and such a confrontational approach is not consistent with wider Swedish cultural norms (Davies 1994).

In sharp contrast, decisions by the German regulatory authorities have been frequently challenged by companies, with a high degree of success. Between 1978 and 1984, there were 362 legal objections to licensing decisions by the German BGA, very often resulting in the granting or partial granting of licences, thus reversing the initial decision by the BGA. For example, in the year between July 1984 and June 1985, there were 95 objections, of which 77 were decided partially or totally in the interest of the objector (Hancher and Reute 1984: 28). In Germany, during the late 1970s and 1980s, the administrative process of drug regulation took place almost entirely within the BGA and was strictly regulated under the Administrative Law, which permits Federal Administrative Courts to publicly examine, challenge and even reverse the actions of civil servants (Anon 1991h: 3). Consequently, the BGA had much less flexibility than many other drug regulatory authorities, and its comparatively formal approach to regulation seems to have led to a more adversarial political culture than in Sweden or the UK. Moreover, the companies' relatively high level of success in judicial review of adverse regulatory decisions is likely to have encouraged further challenges in the courts.

During the late 1980s, as in other countries, the pharmaceutical industry pressed the government and the BGA to accelerate drug approvals. Here again, the courts came into play. In 1987, German companies brought about thirty cases before the Administrative Court against the BGA for 'failing to act' on drug applications. The Court told the BGA that it was obliged to give a decision on an application within 210 days (Anon 1989l). One of these decisions cost the BGA, in effect the state, US$175,000 (Anon 1991h: 2). The Federal Audit Office also drew attention to slow drug approvals at the BGA, which led to the establishment of the division of Central Control within the BGA in 1988. The purpose of the new division was specifically to manage the approval process more 'efficiently' (Anon 1989k). However, the BGA, which received over half of its funding from the central government and about 40 per cent from licensing fees, proved to be much more resistant to industry criticisms than their counterparts in Sweden or the UK.[11] For example, in 1989 staff at the BGA complained publicly that their work was being measured crudely in terms of drug approvals, and that the right-wing coalition government had pushed through amendments to the 1976 German Drug Law in favour of industry at the possible expense of consumer safety, involving the loosening of testing requirements of drugs purportedly offering 'significant therapeutic advances'. It was argued that this was bad for morale within the regulatory agency, because it generated uncertainty among the staff about the purpose of their work (Anon 1989c; Daemmrich 2000).

Senior staff at the regulatory authority also blamed the poor quality of many industry applications for the slow pace of the drug review process (Anon 1989e; Anon 1993l). They asserted that the industry's criticism that the slowness of the BGA in reviewing drug applications was delaying therapeutic advances was not true, because the backlog of applications related to products for which equally good therapeutic alternatives existed on the market. Comparative research on drug regulation tends to support the BGA's view on this matter. In the period 1961 to 1985, more NASs were first introduced in Germany than virtually any other industrialised country, and between 1972 and 1983 NASs reached the market in Germany faster, on average, than in France, Italy, Sweden or the US, but not the UK (Andersson 1992: 62, 68). Moreover, during that period, the FDA estimated that only about half the NCEs approved in the US constituted any therapeutic gain (Dukes 1985: 62). According to Dukes (1985: 23) the longer time taken to market a new drug during the 1980s was heavily influenced by the growing scientific complexity of the chemical and pharmaceutical work involved in new drug development.

Where an application did represent therapeutic advance, according to the BGA delay was due to deficiencies in the application which required additional work to be done by the manufacturer after the approval procedure was under way. Unlike regulatory authorities elsewhere, under German Administrative Law, initially designed to protect the individual against authoritarian government, the BGA could not reject an application found to be deficient before permitting the manufacturer an opportunity to provide the documentation required. Consequently, firms frequently conducted additional work on their applications as the BGA's objections emerged (Anon 1989h).

Of the sixty-two new drugs approved in 1988, only two fell into the BGA's category of 'outstanding significance' (Anon 1989j). This more sceptical view of drug approvals found some support within the German academic community. For example, research at Cologne University found that, of the twenty-six new drugs launched in Germany in 1993, only eight were genuine novelties (Anon 1994c). Nevertheless, drug approval times continued to plague the BGA into the early 1990s, when about 3,000 appeals to the Administrative Court against BGA decisions or 'failures to act' had accumulated. During 1991, the gross mean processing time for 'innovative products' was 920 days, ranging from 30 to 2,100 days. Senior BGA officials noted that the appeals themselves contributed to the lengthy approval times, because once a case went to appeal it might take three years before reaching the Court (Anon 1992f).

The BGA not only had criticisms from the courts and industry with which to contend. While German regulators may have had a reputation for rigour in pre-market checking of new applications, they had been lax in reviewing the efficacy of 'old' drugs which had been left on the market when the AMG 1976 was introduced. As already noted, in the UK the Committee on Review of Medicines was established in 1975 to scrutinise the efficacy of drugs left on the market but never approved under the 1968 Medicines Act. The German equivalent of such a review only began in early 1994 (Anon 1994b; 1995c). Consequently, in 1987 there remained over 155,000 drug products on the German market – the largest in Europe (Hildebrandt 1995b: 909).

Against a background of continued dissatisfaction in industry and government with the BGA's lengthy drug approval times, in 1993 a major 'scandal' broke concerning HIV-infected blood transfusions. Over 350 haemophiliacs had been infected with the HIV virus from blood products (Anon 1993k). The firm which tested the blood products did so using pooled plasma from three donors instead of testing all donations separately, thus cutting costs on test kits but violating the safety procedures set out in law (Anon 1993o). The German Health Minister alleged that the BGA had failed to recognise and react to the problem sufficiently, and vowed to dissolve the regulatory authority, even though the basis for his allegations seemed rather weak (Anon 1993k; Tuffs 1993). He suspended a senior scientist at the BGA, but was forced to reinstate him with different responsibilities because the evidence seemed to exonerate him, although the evidence also suggested that the BGA had handled the matter in an overly legalistic fashion which made the authority slow to act (Anon 1994a; Anon 1995a).

On 1 July 1994, the BGA was disbanded and its work was split between three Federal Institutes under the provisions of the Healthcare Institutions Reform Act: the Federal Institute for Medicinal Products and Devices (Bundesinstitut fur Arzneimittel und Medizinprodukte, or the BfArM), which took over medicines regulation; the Robert Koch Institute, which took over detection, prevention and control of communicable diseases; and the Federal Institute for Consumer Health Protection and Veterinary Medicine, which took over responsibility for the regulation of the safety of food, feedstuffs and veterinary drugs (Zahn 1994). Like the British MCA and the Swedish MPA, the BfArM was formed as a semi-independent regulatory agency following a consultancy report to the government. Previously, at the 'department-oriented' BGA, the director of (human) medicines control reported to more senior staff, such as the President of the BGA, who reported to the Health Minister, but the director of BfArM reports directly to the Minister (Hildebrandt 1995a: 814). Like its British and Swedish counterparts, it also focuses on medicines regulation, but with some 950 staff it is much larger than the MCA or the MPA (Morgenstern 1994).

Significantly, the BfArM retained a government subsidy for 60 per cent of its total budget, needing to derive only 40 per cent from industry fees. According to the director of BfArM, Professor Alfred Hildebrandt, this is not expected to change, because 'it would require a major change in philosophy in Germany'. As he explained: 'It is German policy that drug control is part of the policing laws, and as such you should not pay for the policeman who gives you approval. We come under the funds to protect public health' (Hildebrandt 1995b: 912).

This implies a discernible difference in German regulators' approach to their new status as an independent agency, compared with the stance of their counterparts at the MCA. Underlining this difference in emphasis, Hildebrandt also commented: 'We want not necessarily the fastest assessments, but certainly to produce reliable assessments ... there is a difference between speed, on the one hand, and accuracy of performance, on the other' (1995b: 912).

However, these differences in approach – and, perhaps, sentiment – should not obscure some other fundamental similarities in British and German regulatory reform. These suggest a significant weakening of the resistance to industry criticisms which had been evident within the BGA in the late 1980s. The creation of the BfArM had produced a lot of uncertainty and insecurity among the regulatory staff (Hildebrandt 1995a: 814).

Moreover, in late 1994 the German Ministry of Health warned that BfArM 'could not continue to be so conservative in its approach to the approval of new products' (Anon 1994l: 5). Industry sources argued that the BfArM should

> abandon its apparent principle that all similarly qualified civil servants are infinitely interchangeable with each other, and talk to industry's regulatory affairs staff ... [where] the Ministry would find sufficient consensus on who at the BfArM is competent and who is not, to be able to reorganise the Institute properly.
>
> (Anon 1994l: 5)

Clearly these comments were intended to influence the operation of the BfArM and to change its orientation to one which was more 'market-driven' and responsive to industry interests. At this time, senior regulators adopted the MCA's terminology at the BfArM, where work was organised according to 'business units', which were to set priorities in drug assessments. According to Hildebrandt (1995a), the 'business units' were to be 'customer-oriented', presumably meaning industry-oriented, and they were increasing their efficiency despite increased workload. By 1994, the gross mean approval times had fallen to 684 days, and to about 18 months by 1995 (Zahn 1995).

Furthermore, there are clear signs that industry–regulator relations and consultation have been transformed. Schmitt-Rau (1988: 1065) wrote that 'the German system [of medicines regulation] does not foresee regular discussions between applicant and agency'. According to senior staff at the BfArM, this situation has been changing fast since the mid-1990s. Such changes are acknowledged by industry, whose traditional antagonism to the German regulatory authorities has moderated. Indeed, according to McAuslane (1996), BfArM's approval times, which are much faster than those of the BGA, are among the fastest in Europe.

Under BfArM, some basic regulatory arrangements for new applications remained similar to the situation within the BGA. For example, responsibility for different aspects of drug assessment, such as chemistry, pre-clinical, clinical and pharmacovigilance, continued to rest with different divisions, and relations with the Approval Commissions were not altered. However, the new agency's operational structure gave more emphasis to project group meetings, which cut across different divisions and aimed to reach agreement on an overall assessment of a product's quality, safety and efficacy.[12] As regards 'old' products, whose efficacy had never been demonstrated against the modern standards established since 1976 AMG, the German government extended their 'licences of right' to 2004, despite the potential disadvantages for consumers and patients.[13]

## Conclusion

Burstall (1990: 4) argues that medicines regulation is 'the result of many years of piecemeal action ... determined by the problems, the crises and the misfortunes of the past'. Undoubtedly there is some truth in this, but it also overemphasises medical events at the expense of the compelling roles of organised interests, specifically those of the industry and the state. Prior to the late 1960s, organised consumer interests in the medical field were virtually non-existent in Europe. For example, the oft-cited identification of thalidomide with the genesis of modern drug regulation in Europe is only a half-truth. As we have seen, Sweden's modern pre-market controls were largely in place a quarter of a century before the drug disaster, although post-marketing surveillance was developed as a direct result of thalidomide. Given the insignificant role of organised consumer interests in Sweden at that time, we must conclude that the Swedish state and medical profession gave a much higher priority to public health relative to any conflicting interests derived from the pharmaceutical industry.

Furthermore, the implementation of modern drug regulation lagged behind thalidomide by ten years in the UK and by seventeen years in Germany, even though half-hearted regulatory efforts were introduced within a few years in both countries. The 1968 Medicines Act did not come into force in the UK until 1971 to allow the industry three years to prepare for its implementation, while the AMG 1976 was not implemented until 1978 so that the industry could have two years to adapt to the new drug testing standards expected of it. These developments point to the highly influential role of the pharmaceutical industry in shaping regulation, even in the aftermath of a drug disaster. In both Germany and the UK, governments value the pharmaceutical industry as a national economic asset. This convergence of the commercial interests of the industry and the political interests of the state, combined with the absence of strong organised consumer and public health interests, led to modest, if not weak, beginnings for medicines regulation in Germany and the UK. In 'post-war' Germany, suspicion of strong government agencies also tempered regulatory intervention and motivated the introduction of rigorous Administrative Laws, enabling the regulatory authorities to be readily brought to account in court.

As the regulatory authorities became established, they extended their regulatory activities from the mid-1970s to the mid-1980s – a period often cited as when regulators continually raised pre-market new drug application requirements. Yet even in this period, the industry monopolised access to governmental activities in the field. Industry's access to and consultation with government about medicines regulation was unrivalled by any other interest group in scope and depth. Moreover, the industry maintained a strategic influence over the affairs of medicines regulation via its links with expert scientific advisers. To accommodate this situation, in all three countries, the 'independence' of scientists was given a broad definition so that expert science advisers to the government on the regulation of new drugs could maintain personal and non-personal financial interests in pharmaceutical companies. Relative to other periods of drug regulation, the mid-1970s to the mid-1980s saw a strong nation-state biased towards corporate interests in its representation and planning.

According to Majone (1996: 48–9), across various sectors the rise of 'independent' regulatory agencies is strikingly similar from country to country within the EU. Our research in the pharmaceuticals sector supports this proposition. However, the development of drug regulatory agencies cannot be satisfactorily explained by reference to the 'need for expertise in highly complex and technical matters', 'agencies' separateness from partisan politics' or 'policy continuity' achieved by a relative remoteness from election outcomes. A crucial part of the establishment of drug regulatory agencies has been a neo-liberal political agenda aimed at increasing the responsiveness of regulators to industrial demands at minimal expense to the state. As the state has become more minimal, regulators have become more reliant on consultation and bargaining with industry because, as Peacock (1984: 94–6) makes clear, there is often an inverse relationship between the resources available to the state (for inspection and enforcement) and regulators' need to bargain and negotiate with industry.

This points to the importance of the more general political aims of the state, which defined the terms under which organised interests entered regulatory space. Clear neo-liberal political aims were particularly successful in the absence of any well-formed opposition, although the lack of opposition differed between countries. In Germany, where opposition from regulators was strongest, the influential Administrative Courts provided a formidable ally to the neo-liberal agenda of regulatory reform. The German courts limited the discretion of regulators to impose strict but time-consuming checks on industry's new drugs. In Sweden, a more consensual culture militated against companies making significant use of the courts, but that same culture also meant that regulators opposed to the neo-liberal regulatory reforms found little base of support in the wider professional and consumer communities. Meanwhile, in the UK the flexible style of British regulatory culture encouraged officials to embrace a neo-liberal agenda for regulatory policy. Although opposition from consumer and public health advocacy groups was better organised in the UK than Germany or Sweden, it had very limited success against a well-oiled government–industry alliance.

While differences between medicines regulation in the three countries certainly exist, our most striking finding is the similarity in trajectory since the late 1980s. In all three countries, the political interests of the state have shifted towards neo-liberalism. The large extent to which the Swedish and German governments have followed the British approach to the establishment of a drug regulatory agency provides support for the theory of 'early' and 'late' regulators. Since the late 1980s, it does seem to be the case that the way the UK government set up the MCA has become a model for other EU countries following later along the regulatory road.

Despite the much more organised consumer interests in this period, they have been no match for the combined power of industry and political interests, even in Germany and Sweden where regulators expressed scepticism, if not downright opposition, to the implication of neo-liberal policies for the protection of public health. In Germany, regulatory reform has been more resistant to neo-liberal developments, probably because the regulators have retained much of their financial independence from industry fees, and hence job security. Indeed, during the 1980s and 1990s, the industry complained not only that the BGA took too long to approve drugs, but also that it was hostile to industry. Nevertheless, the evidence from our research and beyond suggests that the regulatory authorities in all three countries have responded to industrial concerns by reducing regulatory review times for NASs in recent years, and by increasing consultation with manufacturers. Modern national drug regulation is not a proxy for medical accidents and the misfortunes of drug disasters but, above all, a product of the state's negotiation with, and accommodation of, organised industrial interests.

# Chapter 4

# The Europeanisation of medicines regulation

In this chapter, we explain why the research-based pharmaceutical industry wants European, and indeed global, harmonisation of medicines regulation. These industrial interests are strong supporters of a single European market for pharmaceuticals and exert considerable influence on the regulatory regime in Europe. We also trace the origins of the Europeanisation of medicines regulation, and discuss the gradual development of the 'weak' European regulatory state from 1975 to 1995. This period saw the establishment of a body of expert scientists, known as the Committee for Proprietary Medicinal Products (CPMP). In particular, we examine why that 'weak' European regulatory state failed to achieve European harmonisation, and how it was supplanted by a 'strong' regulatory state in 1995, with the establishment of the European Agency for the Evaluation of Medicinal Products (EMEA) and binding arbitration to settle disputes between Member States of the EU. The EMEA, together with other supranational regulatory institutions such as the CPMP and the Commission, attained greater authority over both national regulatory agencies and the industry. This 'efficiency regime' requires Member States to mutually recognise each other's assessments and marketing approval recommendations much more readily and quickly. Finally, we discuss efforts to harmonise procedures for monitoring the safety of medicines already on the market: that is, pharmacovigilance, an area that remains relatively underdeveloped within the overall harmonisation project in Europe.

## The industry's transnational agenda

As we discussed in Chapter 3, for several decades European industry associations have badgered their national governments and regulatory agencies to organise medicines regulation according to their desire for fast approvals. However, the industry's products are marketed on a worldwide scale, and increasingly industry has adopted a 'global outlook' to regulatory issues, a trend which is itself linked to growing procedural and technical harmonisation. Over half of the sales of the fifty largest companies are made outside their 'home country' (Vogel 1998: 1).

Industry interest in developing a global strategy stems from political pressure to reduce health costs combined with continuing regulatory demands, both of which contribute to longer development times and shorter product lifecycles. A shorter 'time to approval' translates into a quicker return on investment. European and global harmonisation helps to achieve this goal because more markets can be accessed more or less simultaneously, in theory at least. Conversely, separate and distinct national regulatory regimes, with different technical standards and divergent safety regulations, add to the costs of transnational companies. To this extent, industry interests converge with those of the Commission and national governments, which are committed to greater economic integration.

Government officials at the European Commission did not need much convincing of the virtues of harmonisation. For example, Cecchini, who wrote a Commission report on the European Single Market, accepted the argument put forward by the European pharmaceutical industry that it was significantly constrained by the 'lengthy and differing drug registration procedures' of the EU Member States (Cecchini 1988, cited in Vogel 1998: 1, 4). Similarly, in 1995, the European Commissioner noted that during the previous twenty years the EU's share of all new medicines developed had declined from a half to a third, while the US held four times as many patents in the biotechnology sector as the EU. Against this background, as Vogel (1998: 5) notes:

> An important objective of the creation of a single European drug approval procedure was to promote more European-wide drug research and development, thus helping the industry to confidently continue to hold its place on the world stage in the foreseeable future.

Yet across the Atlantic, numerous researchers and policy

analysts held the FDA's more stringent regulatory posture towards industry in the 1970s and 1980s responsible for reduced productivity of drug R and D in the US (Dukes 1985: 39–41). This suggests that the identification of regulation as the culprit for the limited fortunes of pharmaceutical R and D in the EU may well have been a crude oversimplification. Other factors are likely to have been important, such as the expiry of important patents for products developed in the post-war 'golden age' of drug discovery; the growing technical complexity and cost of innovative research; and the increased sophistication and influence of generic manufacturing companies.

Not surprisingly, the industry has organised its interest representation to reflect its transnational priorities, although it was not until 1978 that the European Federation of Pharmaceutical Industry Associations (EFPIA), comprising the national industry associations, was established as the official representative of the European industry in negotiations with the Commission, the European Parliament and the CPMP. In formal terms, each national association adopts a national position, which is then passed to the European level represented by EFPIA. Most importantly, EFPIA represents industry in the consultation process over proposed EU legislation, changes in marketing authorisation procedures, and technical guidelines on drug testing and monitoring. However, in practice some of the more powerful firms lobby EFPIA directly, or even the EMEA, bypassing their national associations. To reflect conflicting interests within the industry, EFPIA reorganised its structure in 1997, allowing the large research-based companies full membership, along with the sixteen national associations, plus associate status for smaller firms (Anon 1997m). The trend for transnational firms to attempt to influence policy directly at the European level again reflects increasing globalisation, making it difficult to identify specifically national or European companies (Wyatt-Walter 1995). By the mid-1980s, the industry had established a European 'regulatory group', aiming to: submit the same core application to every country; minimise approval times, especially the time between first and last approval; and ensure approvals were consistent with the company's labelling requirements (Barrowcliffe 1996). One senior industry official summarised the strategy as 'to have the easiest, fastest, and most uniform [regulatory] assessment route across Europe'.[1]

## Legal instruments for harmonisation

There have been numerous initiatives over the past thirty years aimed at harmonising legal, scientific and administrative procedures governing the sale of medicinal products in the EU, with the pace of change particularly rapid during the 1990s.[2] These initiatives can conveniently be split into two types: scientific (chemical and pharmaceutical data, pre-clinical tests, clinical studies), and administrative (procedures and practices required for registration). The overall process of European harmonisation can be viewed according to these two dimensions: the harmonisation of technical requirements, and procedural harmonisation, though this is *not* to suggest that the two are entirely separate.

EU legislative activity can take several forms: Directives, Regulations, Council Decisions, Recommendations, proposals and so on and so forth. Each of these mechanisms is important, but Directives, which can emanate from the Council of Ministers or the Commission, rank as the most significant tool because they provide the foundation for all other activity, such as additional legislation (e.g. Regulations) or Commission guidelines (officially known as Communications). Above all, the key Directives define the scientific, technical and administrative requirements to be met and the procedural rules to be followed before a marketing authorisation is granted.[3]

The regulation of pharmaceuticals in Europe has developed within the familiar dualistic 'regulator/sponsor' framework, whereby regulators are charged with both ensuring the safety and efficacy of medicines and promoting the industry's well-being. This approach is now firmly embedded in European law. According to the Commission, EU medicines legislation has consistently pursued two objectives: the protection of public health and the free movement of products. Ostensibly, these two principles underlie the entire harmonisation process in Europe (European Commission 1989; European Commission 1994: 1; MCA 1993a). Thus, the first of the so-called 'framework directives' (Directive 65/65/EEC) opens by stating:

> The primary purpose of any rules concerning the production and distribution of medicinal products must be to safeguard public health ... however this objective must be attained by means which will not hinder the development of the

pharmaceutical industry or trade in medicinal products within the Community.

(European Commission 1965; European Commission 1995: 35)[4]

Three Council Directives, in particular, provide the legal bedrock upon which European harmonisation is built.[5] Directive 65/65/EEC stipulates that no product can be placed on the market of a Member State unless a marketing authorisation has been issued by the competent authorities of the Member State, in accordance with the Directive, and lists the scientific and administrative documentation an applicant must provide.[6] Ten years later, Directive 75/318/EEC provided the framework of analytical, pharmaco-toxicological and clinical standards and protocols for testing medicinal products. While Directive 75/318/EEC extended the framework provided in 65/65/EEC by setting out the particular requirements relating to applications, including the qualifications and roles of experts and the assessment of the product dossier, Directive 75/319/EEC also established the first EU authorisation procedure based on the mutual recognition of national assessments (the so-called 'CPMP procedure') and, crucially, established the CPMP 'to facilitate the adoption of a common position by the Member States with regard to decisions on the issuing of marketing authorisations' (European Commission 1975a, 1975b).

Directives 65/65/EEC and 75/319/EEC, in particular, went a considerable way towards harmonising existing national approval systems while providing the foundation for future initiatives, and the second provided the basis for enforcing European-wide technical standards. The early stages of harmonisation were therefore characterised by a gradual alignment of national rules and procedures, achieved to a greater or lesser degree according to the Member State. This occurred under the aegis of these three 'framework' Directives, along with a large number of technical guidelines, many of which arose from existing national guidelines (Jones and Jefferys 1994; Jefferys and Jones 1995).

An important second phase of legislation in the 1980s amended these original Directives in several ways. Directive 83/570/EEC introduced a simplified mutual recognition approval procedure (the 'multi-state procedure'), while Directive 87/22/EEC set up the so-called 'concertation procedure', a process of concertation between the Commission and Member States before any national decision was taken on the registration of 'high technology products', especially those derived from biotechnology 'with a view to arriving at uniform decisions throughout the Community' on such products (European Commission 1983, 1987). However, as discussed below, both procedures failed to fulfil expectations, although the latter was more successful in terms of applications submitted and agreements over labelling, known as the summary of product characteristics (Jones and Jefferys 1994). Both were subsequently modified by further legislation aimed at speeding up approvals and encouraging companies to use specifically European procedures.

Overall, there have been three procedures to date for the mutual recognition of marketing authorisations by Member States: the 'CPMP procedure', which operated from 1976 to 1985; the 'multi-state procedure', in place from 1985 to 1995; and the 'decentralised procedure' (or simply 'mutual recognition procedure', as it is increasingly called), introduced in 1995. The first two, which were very similar in content, constituted what we characterise as the 'weak' European regulatory state, while the latter constitutes (along with the centralised procedure for biotechnology and other innovative products introduced at the same time) the 'strong' regulatory state. Together, these developments signal implementation of a new 'efficiency regime' for pharmaceuticals in Europe.

## Mutual recognition: the CPMP procedure

The CPMP procedure, established by Council Directive 75/319/EEC and implemented in November 1976, allowed a company which obtained a marketing authorisation in one Member State to apply for approval simultaneously in at least five other Member States, by asking the authorising Member State to forward a copy of the first evaluation to the other countries. But the procedure was not popular with industry. Only 41 applications were made in the eight years it operated, and these were mostly for generic or 'me-too' products, rather than NASs. Of the 41 applications, 28 (70 per cent) received a favourable opinion; the remaining 13 (30 per cent) received an unfavourable opinion, of which 5 were unanimous. The 41 applications led to 175 authorisations and 65 final refusals (i.e. refusals after all national appeal stages) (Cartwright and Matthews 1991). Because of industry dissatisfaction, the procedure was modified in 1985 to permit applicants to use the initial approval to apply to two or more rather than at least five other Member States. The new procedure, known as the 'multi-state procedure', also allowed applicants direct access to the CPMP in the event of a dispute (a right which was not available under some Member States' national procedures) (European Commission 1983).

## Mutual recognition: the multi-state procedure

One of the reasons we might expect industry to welcome mutual recognition is because it allows companies to submit applications without the need for regulatory staff in every country concerned, reducing costs and (possibly) speeding up the approval process. Despite this, most companies failed to use the multi-state procedure to any great extent, although the number of applications did increase somewhat towards the end of the 1980s, as companies sought to gain experience prior to introduction of the decentralised procedure in 1995. Evidence also shows that the procedure was initially used mainly by smaller companies, which could benefit most from regulatory 'economies of scale', often in order to 'sell on' a first authorisation to a local licensee or distributor in other Member States. Certain firms used the procedure to circumvent delays in national registration procedures, since if a Member State did not submit 'reasoned objections' within 120 days of the first authorisation, it had to accept the original authorisation. Some transnational companies refused to use the procedure at all, while others adopted a more sophisticated approach, using the procedure to accelerate approvals by filing several national applications and then withdrawing them if there were delays, which was a legitimate strategy. Once approval was obtained in one Member State, the company would then use the procedure to progress authorisations in the other countries. Also, comparatively few applications were for NASs. Some national authorities took the view that the procedure should be used mainly for innovative products and not for 'me-too' or second applicant products with no particular therapeutic advantage. In such cases, they were unwilling to act as rapporteur, as the country of first approval was then called, particularly if they had only limited resources.

The countries for which authorisation is sought based on an existing approval in another Member State are known as the Concerned Member States. An interesting feature during the period prior to 1995 was that the average number of Concerned Member States involved in applications grew, despite the reduction in the number of Member States required to use the procedure after 1985. Overall, however, industry's experience of the procedure was that it was slow, bureaucratic and, *above all, ineffective in terms of Member States recognising a first approval.* In other words, national regulatory agencies did not mutually recognise each other's assessments of applications in terms of safety and/or efficacy evaluation, or perhaps on other criteria. Companies therefore remained generally sceptical of the advantages of the multi-state procedure, and the great majority of applications prior to introduction of the decentralised procedure in 1995 were submitted via national approval routes.[7]

This led the Commission to search for ways of encouraging companies to use mutual recognition and force Member States to recognise other countries' assessments. Legally, Article 9(1) of Directive 75/319/EEC directed national authorities to take 'due consideration' of the marketing authorisation of another Member State. This did not mean, however, that mutual recognition was automatic because the same active ingredient is often contained in different products across the EU. The assessment report compiled by the originating (rapporteur) authority simply provided other national agencies with information on the issues which the first authority had considered during its assessment, including questions raised with the applicant and responses given (Cartwright and Matthews 1991: 169). As we shall see below, what has happened over time is the erosion of the right of Member States to conduct assessments at the speed they wish, and ultimately to reject a product if in their view it does not meet local standards for quality, safety and efficacy.

## The industry's blueprint for Europe

Conscious of the failings of the multi-state procedure, in 1988 the industry set out its preferred system for Europeanised medicines regulation in the form of the ABPI's 'Blueprint for Europe'. The ABPI stressed that the most important condition for industry was that companies should be able to obtain a single, uniform marketing authorisation, based on a clear set of data requirements and issued within 210 days. They proposed that a centralised EU drug regulatory authority (not the CPMP) should handle all biotechnology products directly, while companies could retain the option of submitting non-biotechnological, innovative products either to the decentralised EU authority or to national authorities within a mutual recognition procedure. All non-biotechnological and non-innovative products would be processed within the mutual recognition procedure. Under the proposed mutual recognition procedure, if national regulatory agencies failed to mutually recognise each other's assessments within a specified period, then the EU drug regulatory authority could *impose* a decision on the Member States (Anon 1988d: 7).

## Mutual recognition: the decentralised procedure

Industry's refusal to utilise the multi-state procedure to any great extent, combined with the Commission's commitment to greater harmonisation, led to the replacement of the multi-state procedure in 1995. Since January 1995, a company wishing to market a product in more than one Member State has been able to seek authorisation in other Member States by a revamped mutual recognition procedure known as the decentralised (or, as it is often called, mutual recognition) procedure. Like its predecessor, this is achieved by asking two or more Member States to recognise the marketing authorisation granted by the Member State of first approval – the so-called Reference Member State – within 90 days. Equally, Member States can initiate the process, even in cases where the company has not requested mutual recognition (European Commission 1996a: 7).

The decentralised procedure is in effect an extension of the former multi-state procedure, since regulatory approval is based on the mutual recognition of an existing authorisation. However, there are a number of highly significant changes, which together mark the turning point from the 'weak' to the 'strong' European regulatory state. The major new provision is that disagreements between Member States *must* now be resolved at the EU level under the auspices of the EMEA's scientific committee, the CPMP; and, crucially, the outcome is *binding on the Member States concerned*. This is the defining difference between the multi-state procedure and the decentralised procedure. Furthermore, since 1998, the procedure has been mandatory for all products, except those submitted via the centralised procedure (see below), homeo-pathic products, those (relatively few) products intended to be marketed only in a single country, and generics, in which case local authorisation is still possible.[8] Hence, where a product has been approved in one Member State, any application to market the same product in other EU countries will *automatically* be subject to mutual recognition (plus arbitration in the event of a dispute). A pictorial presentation of the new system, including timeframes, is given in Figure 4.1.

Strict time limits are prescribed for the procedure as a whole, with 120 days for initial evaluation and 90 days for consultation with concerned Member States (the so-called 'clarification and dialogue' period). Although the timetable is not legally enforceable, because national agencies now compete for business (industry fees), Member States are under intense pressure to conform. Time and again, industry representatives confirmed that they look for fast approval rates, coupled with high-quality assessments, when determining company authorisation strategy. There is also substantial evidence that regulatory agencies have been forced to reduce assessment times in order to meet the new timetables. Acquiescence in industry's demand for ever faster approvals, along with reduced assessment times brought about by the new regulatory structures and inter-agency competition, are key features of the new 'efficiency regime' in Europe. It is also clear that the Europeanised system of mutual recognition finally adopted by the Commission very closely resembles the 'blueprint' proposed by industry, except that the CPMP has retained its central role as the EU's expert drug regulatory authority, albeit supported by the EMEA.

As with the multi-state procedure, mutual recognition under the decentralised procedure is not automatic. Nevertheless, under the new system a marketing authorisation granted by one Member State ought to be recognised 'in principle' by other Member States unless there are 'grounds for supposing that the authorisation ... may present a risk to public health'. Clearly, defining what constitutes a 'risk to public health' is open to debate and, potentially, serious disagreement between Member States. Officially, the expression simply refers to the three standard regulatory criteria for pharmaceuticals: quality, safety and efficacy (European Commission 1996a: 7).

In practice, if a Member State refuses to accept an authorisation from another Member State, it must immediately inform the company, the Reference Member State, the other Concerned Member

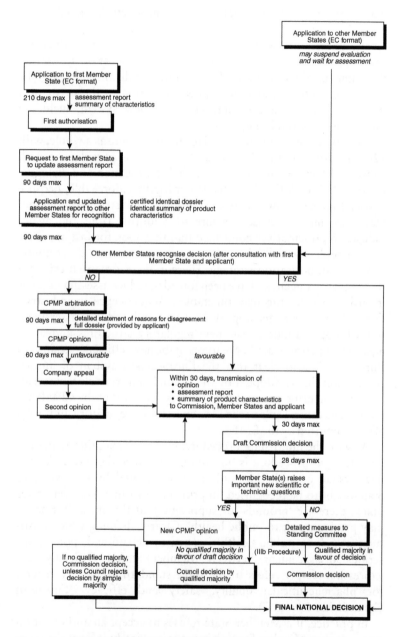

*Figure 4.1*   The EU's decentralised procedure for marketing
authorisation of new drugs

States, and the CPMP, stating the reasons for its decision and indicating how the gaps in the application might be filled. A compulsory conciliation stage follows within the 90-day period allowed for Member States to recognise the original approval (Deboyser 1996b: 117). This arrangement puts regulators under considerable pressure to quickly adopt a position on the original authorisation and to assemble evidence in support of their own position if they propose to reject it. In another effort to reduce delays and encourage agreement among Member States, the Commission has also restricted the subjects on which Concerned Member States can raise queries during the 'dialogue phase' (i.e. the period immediately after the initial assessment) to four areas: indications, dosage and method of administration, contra-indications, and shelf-life and storage requirements.

The detailed procedure followed depends upon whether it is a Member State or a company which initiates mutual recognition. If a Member State initiates the procedure, other Member States can suspend detailed examination of the application in order to await the assessment being prepared by the other Member States. According to the Commission, this rule was introduced to allow efficient utilisation of resources and avoid duplication of effort. Within 90 days of receipt of the assessment report, the Concerned Member State is normally obliged to recognise the decision of the Reference Member State and accept the approved summary of product characteristics by granting a marketing authorisation with an identical summary of product characteristics, or, in the case of a negative assessment, by refusing the application, in which case the matter is referred to the CPMP for arbitration, which we discuss below (European Commission 1996a: 10).

Companies can also withdraw an application at any time during the procedure, except at the arbitration stage. The benefit for a company is that it may want to withdraw an application from one (or more) countries for commercial reasons, or because it perceives that a particular Member State is likely to reject aspects of the application, such as a claimed indication. Withdrawing a decentralised application from a 'tough' Member State removes that agency from discussions on the proposed summary of product characteristics and also any subsequent CPMP deliberations, thereby protecting the company's investment in the product. This 'escape route' has been widely used. Until 1998, any 'excluded' application could then be handled on a national basis, although this option is no longer available with the end of national licensing. On the other hand, companies need to tread carefully in this area because Member States may look unfavourably on partial withdrawals (i.e. from one or more Member States), and the strategy may actually encourage increased scrutiny by the remaining Member States. The German regulatory agency, for example, has publicly announced that it will automatically send withdrawn products to arbitration, and the Commission has threatened similar action (Anon 1996f). Details about the number of applications submitted via the decentralised (mutual recognition) procedure since its introduction in 1995, and the Reference Member States (RMSs) used, are provided in Tables 4.1 to 4.3.

Overall, the post-1995 mutual recognition procedure is a hybrid system: while still based on national marketing authorisations, it establishes relationships between these national authorisations

Table 4.1   Number of finalised mutual recognition (decentralised) procedures (1995 to June 1999)

|                    | 1995 | 1996 | 1997 | 1998 | June 1999 |
|--------------------|------|------|------|------|-----------|
| NAS                | 5    | 32   | 40   | 37   | 11        |
| Others             | 2    | 19   | 34   | 42   | 18        |
| Generics, OTC, etc.| 3    | 36   | 69   | 103  | 29        |
| Total*             | 10   | 87   | 143  | 182  | 58        |

Source:   MRFG (http://heads.medagencies.org/mrfg)
Note:   *includes double and triple procedures (N = 480)

Table 4.2   Total number of finalised mutual recognition (decentralised) procedures by type* (1995 to June 1999)

| Type of substance              | N   | %    |
|--------------------------------|-----|------|
| New active substances (NASs)   | 125 | 26   |
| Others                         | 115 | 23.9 |
| Generics                       | 113 | 23.5 |
| Line extension                 | 64  | 13.3 |
| Fixed combination              | 46  | 9.6  |
| OTC                            | 13  | 2.7  |
| Herbal                         | 3   | 0.7  |
| Blood products                 | 1   | 0.3  |

Source:   MRFG (http://heads.medagencies.org/mrfg)
Note:   * number includes double and triple procedures (N = 480)

Table 4.3    Percentage of procedures per Reference Member State
(NASs) 1995 to June 1999*

| Reference Member State | % |
|---|---|
| Austria | 0 |
| Belgium | 0 |
| Denmark | 1 |
| Finland | 3 |
| France | 18 |
| Germany | 15 |
| Greece | 0 |
| Ireland | 1 |
| Italy | 1 |
| Luxembourg | 0 |
| Netherlands | 12 |
| Portugal | 0 |
| Spain | 1 |
| Sweden | 19 |
| United Kingdom | 29 |

Source:   MRFG (http://heads.medagencies.org/mrfg)
Note:   *includes double and triple NAS procedures (N = 135)

granted under the procedure such that they can only be amended,
suspended or withdrawn on the basis of decisions taken by the EU
as a whole. If Member States object to a first authorisation, the
dispute is resolved by arbitration through the CPMP at the
European level.

## CPMP arbitration

The arbitration of disputes between Member States arising in the
decentralised procedure is one of the tasks of the CPMP, as laid
down in Directive 75/319/EEC. The CPMP is the scientific advisory
committee of the EMEA and comprises representatives from each
of the fifteen Member States, plus the Commission. Previously
appointed to 'represent' Member States, these are now officially
appointed as 'individuals' based on scientific merit. Basically,

arbitration is possible in three situations: when a Member State refuses to recognise another Member State's authorisation; in order to harmonise divergent decisions among Member States, such as whether to license a product; and where 'Community interests' are claimed to be involved, in which case either Member States, the Commission or an applicant may refer a matter to the CPMP (European Commission 1975b).[9]

When a marketing authorisation is granted by a Member State (that is, the Reference Member State), other concerned Member States (that is, the Concerned Member States) to which an application for mutual recognition has been made are required to recognise the authorisation within a period of 90 days. Likewise, a Member State suspending the evaluation of a national application in order to await the assessment report of a Member State, which has already authorised or is evaluating the same product, is also required to recognise the first approval within 90 days. Where one or more Concerned Member States are not able to recognise the decision of the Reference Member State on the grounds that this would 'present a risk to public health', as permitted under Article 7(2) of Directive 65/65/EEC, Member States are first required to seek agreement among themselves (European Commission 1965). When agreement cannot be reached, the matter is referred to the CPMP for arbitration. Once adopted, the CPMP opinion, and the resulting summary of product characteristics, is enforced through a binding Commission decision. The CPMP has 90 days to consult and express a recommendation, and is free to consider other public health questions besides those addressed by the referring Member State(s) (EMEA 1996a). As with a centralised application, the CPMP appoints a rapporteur for the referral and/or can call on individual experts for specific questions, and the overall process is overseen by a project manager appointed by the EMEA.

The arbitration procedure is also used if a Member State considers it necessary, for public health reasons, to amend, suspend or withdraw an existing authorisation (i.e. a product already on the market). In this case, the procedure is automatically initiated by the Member State concerned, without prior consultation with other Member States which have also authorised the product.[10] Until a final decision is reached, any country may 'exceptionally, suspend the marketing and use of the medical product concerned on its territory, setting out the emergency and public health grounds that warrant the step' (Deboyser 1996b: 121).

Thus another novel feature of the mutual recognition procedure is that despite Member States' support for mutual recognition, demonstrated by the passing of Directive 93/39/EEC, an individual Member State can still refuse to recognise another Member State's authorisation and thereby force the EU as a whole to take a decision, with which all Member States must then comply. A corollary of this is that the arbitration procedure can lead to a negative decision on the product concerned, with the existing authorisation in one or more Member States being amended, suspended or even withdrawn completely (Deboyser 1996b: 121).

The introduction of the multi-state procedure did little to reduce disputes between Member States, with all but one authorisation granted under the procedure being referred to the CPMP. By contrast, since the start of the decentralised procedure and binding arbitration in January 1995, there have been comparatively very few arbitration cases. Only three referrals had occurred by the end of 1996, with a total of six final opinions issued by the CPMP by June 1999.[11]

The first of these was initiated by Hoechst AG, and centred on the refusal of Austria and Portugal to recognise a first approval granted by the Netherlands for Amaryl, an oral diabetes treatment. Besides being the first arbitration under the new rules, what was also significant was that the company was supported by at least one national agency, the Swedish MPA, and probably by others, in its decision to seek arbitration. Both the company and the MPA argued that the objecting Member States had interpreted the significance of liver tumours in rats incorrectly, according to the latest carcinogenicity science and extrapolation techniques. As well as believing it had a good case (the product was already approved in Sweden, the Netherlands and the USA), the company was encouraged to go to arbitration because both company and regulators were unsure how the process would operate in practice. In other words, in seeking the opinion of the CPMP, Hoechst saw themselves as testing the procedure in a more general sense on behalf of both industry and regulatory authorities.[12] The CPMP eventually recommended authorisation, with amendments to the summary of product characteristics, and this was converted into a Decision by the Commission in August 1996 (EMEA 1998c).

It is not self-evident from the official discourse why the situation has been transformed from one where virtually all applications for mutual recognition before 1995 ended in arbitration, while Member

States have been able to reach agreement without arbitration subsequently. One might conclude that the introduction of binding arbitration has forced Member States to discard their own 'national interests' and accept EU decisions. Yet, according to Member States' own pronouncements, earlier disputes were founded on scientific disagreements, just as post-1995 ones presumably are. This suggests that what are essentially administrative changes (introduction of binding opinions, greater contact between agency officials) have effectively suppressed medical–scientific disputes in the new 'efficiency' regime.

## The concertation procedure

Separate procedures for biotechnology and other 'high-tech' products, including NASs, have been in force since 1987. However, as with mutual recognition, we can identify two stages in the development of European procedures for such products: the concertation procedure introduced in July 1987, and the centralised procedure introduced in January 1995 (European Commission 1987).

The concertation procedure provided a simple Community-wide licensing opinion on biotechnology products, for which it was mandatory, before individual national licensing decisions were made. It was also an option for so-called 'high technology' products, when the applicant could justify use of the procedure. Concertation was automatically triggered once a competent authority received an application for a biotechnology product (as defined in List A of the Annex to Directive 87/22/EEC). 'High tech' (innovative) products (defined in List B of the same Annex) included products for an entirely new indication; those administered by a new innovative delivery system; and those manufactured by a new technique or significant advancement (European Commission 1987).

Under the procedure, a product was assessed by a Member State (the 'rapporteur') on behalf of the EU as a whole, though the company was obliged to send a summary of the dossier and the expert reports to all other Member States. The rapporteur made a detailed assessment of the dossier and circulated its assessment report and recommendations to other Member States. It is reasonable to assume that, in practice, the other concerned authorities also undertook at least a partial review. Comments and concerns were fed back to the rapporteur, who sent them to the manufacturer and, in turn, assessed the company's responses. 'Reasoned objections' were submitted by Member States to the CPMP for discussion. If approved by the CPMP, marketing authorisation was then permissible in all Member States and the procedure, in theory at least, gave the applicant what was effectively a European licence. However, *like the multi-state procedure, CPMP opinions were non-binding* and Member States could, if they wished, approve or reject applications without reference to the CPMP opinion.

By 1994, about fifty products had entered the concertation procedure, and for most of them Member States agreed a common summary of product characteristics across the EU (Jones and Jefferys 1994). The UK MCA was the lead agency in around half the applications (MCA 1993b). From this perspective, the procedure was more successful than the multi-state procedure since the CPMP was able to reach uniform and positive opinions, which were translated into consistent national approvals, although national variations remained.

## The centralised procedure

The centralised procedure, which replaced the concertation procedure on 1 January 1995, is essentially an extension of the earlier procedure. Like its predecessor, the new procedure is mandatory for products derived from biotechnology and optional for other innovatory products, including NASs and products derived from human blood or plasma. The CPMP decides whether a product comes under the latter category: that is, whether it is innovatory (so-called List B products) (European Commission 1993a: Annex). The official reason for restricting access to certain types of product is that it was necessary to introduce the new structures gradually, and to ensure a smooth transfer of responsibility for 'centralised' products from Member States to the EU, although in practice the number of NASs accepted has increased rapidly (Deboyser 1996a). Details of centralised applications submitted between 1995 and June 1999 are shown in Table 4.4.

Assessment under the procedure is through a single application to the EMEA. If the application is approved, the outcome is a single authorisation allowing access to the market in all Member States. As with mutual recognition, the key difference compared to the concertation procedure is that *the opinion of the CPMP is now binding on all Member States* (European Commission 1993a; European Commission 1996a: 31–49). Second, unlike the concertation

*Table 4.4*    Number of centralised procedures 1995 to 1999[*]

| | 1995–1998 | | | 1999 (to June) | | | Overall Total |
|---|---|---|---|---|---|---|---|
| | Part A | Part B | Total | Part A | Part B | Total | |
| Applications submitted | 62 | 115 | 177 | 12 | 13 | 25 | 202 |
| Withdrawals | 11 | 19 | 30 | 1 | 5 | 6 | 36 |
| Positive CPMP opinions | 35 | 65 | 100 | 6 | 13 | 19 | 119[1] |
| Negative CPMP opinions[2] | 1 | 2 | 3 | 0 | 0 | 0 | 3[3] |
| Marketing authorisations granted by the Commission | 28 | 60 | 88 | 9 | 11 | 20 | 108[4] |

*Source:*    EMEA 1999c: 5

*Notes:*
[*] excludes variations and extensions
[1] 119 opinions corresponding to 93 substances
[2] in case of appeal the opinion is not counted again
[3] negative opinions corresponding to 2 substances
[4] 108 marketing authorisations corresponding to 84 substances

procedure, the applicant can no longer choose the evaluating Member State, although they are encouraged to state their preferences.

The first product authorised under the centralised procedure was Ares-Serono's anti-fertility treatment, Gonal-F in October 1995.[13] By early 1996, the Agency had received 30 new applications under the centralised procedure consisting of 9 under Part A and 21 under Part B of the Annex to Regulation (EEC) 2309/93, signifying that two-thirds of applicants were voluntarily using the centralised procedure, a figure which has been maintained (EMEA 1996e; Anon 1996c; EMEA 1999g).[14] By June 1999, there had been a total of 198 applications submitted via the EMEA route, with 116 positive and 3 negative CPMP opinions resulting. Of the positive opinions, 106 had been converted into marketing authorisations by the Commission, corresponding to 82 substances. The Committee has also given an opinion on nearly 600 variations to existing authorisations since 1995 (EMEA 1999c).

Withdrawal is possible before the CPMP issues an opinion. Recently, the EMEA has become increasingly concerned about the rising number of withdrawals (35 since 1995, around 22 per cent) and, as a result, created a Working Group on Withdrawn Applications to analyse the phenomenon (EMEA 1999d). A preliminary analysis of 30 product withdrawals to 1998 identified inadequate development or premature data in the case of 7 products (23 per cent), methodological concerns connected with efficacy in the case of 14 products (43 per cent), while 11 products (37 per cent) showed inadequate therapeutic effect. Safety concerns were identified with 15 products (50 per cent). The study found that companies mainly withdraw applications at Day 120, i.e. on receiving the List of Questions from the CPMP, with smaller numbers withdrawing at later points in the process (EMEA 1999e: 6).

## The timetable for centralised evaluations

Once an application is validated and the dossier received, the evaluation procedure starts. The EMEA appoints a project manager for each application, but during the course of assessment the applicant may liaise directly with the rapporteur for clarification of specific issues relating to the data submitted, and inform the project manager of the outcome. The total time permitted for arriving at an opinion under the centralised procedure is 210 days, which is broken down as follows: the rapporteur and co-rapporteur have 70 days to produce the preliminary assessment report, which is forwarded to CPMP members and also sent to the applicant. During the next 50 days, the CPMP considers the assessment report(s) produced by the rapporteur and co-rapporteur; comments are exchanged between CPMP members, the EMEA, and the (co-)rapporteurs; and a list of outstanding questions is drawn up and sent with 'short provisional conclusions' to the applicant (European Commission 1996a: 43).

This 'Summary of Conclusions' states whether the product is approvable providing satisfactory answers are given to questions and/or specific changes are made (e.g. to the indications or the summary of product characteristics). When the company responds to any questions, the 'clock' is started again. The deadline for comments from CPMP members to (co-)rapporteur(s) on the company's response is 170 days, and the CPMP is obliged to reach an opinion and produce a draft assessment report by day 210. If oral presentations to the CPMP are required, the clock is stopped to allow preparation of these. Before day 240 the CPMP 'Report and Opinion' is finalised and transmitted to the applicant, the Commission and Member States in all EU languages. The last CPMP stage is the finalisation of the European Public Assessment Report (EPAR) in consultation with the company and the (co-) rapporteur(s), which occurs before day 300 (European Commission 1996a: 43). The EPARs, which are discussed further in Chapter 7, are publicly available summaries of the CPMP's regulatory assessment of individual products approved.

The draft opinion is prepared by the secretariat and then adopted by the CPMP. Officially, the Committee's opinion, which may be favourable or unfavourable, is

> wherever possible reached by scientific consensus. Where a scientific consensus cannot be obtained, the majority position is given as the opinion, with divergent positions and the reasons for such positions being included at the request of the members concerned.
>
> (European Commission 1996a: 46)

The final assessment report and the final summary of product characteristics are prepared by the rapporteur and co-rapporteur, in co-ordination with the project manager, 'taking account of the full scientific debate with the Committee and the conclusions reached' (ibid.). Once adopted, this becomes the CPMP assessment report and is appended to the Committee's opinion, which also includes the proposed summary of product characteristics, and where appropriate divergent positions of members.

The applicant can appeal against the opinion if it does not accept the amendments and/or conditions imposed. Otherwise, the EMEA forwards the opinion within 30 days to the Commission, the Member States and the applicant, together with the assessment report. In other words, if no appeal is lodged, it is assumed that the opinion is accepted. The time taken to assess a product in the centralised procedure currently varies between 169 and 189 days, with an additional 32 to 45 day post-opinion phase (EMEA 1999g). The Commission prepares a draft authorisation, based on the CPMP opinion, which must be approved by the Standing Committee, a 'quasi-political' committee comprising representatives from each Member State. Formally, the Standing Committee cannot re-open questions within the provenance of the CPMP – that is 'scientific' issues – and normally accepts proposed authorisations. Nonetheless, the Standing Committee is potentially very powerful because its approval marks the final stage in the centralised procedure and because it can return recommendations to the CPMP for further consideration. If the draft authorisation is accepted, the Commission then produces the final authorisation documents. Once granted, the authorisation is valid for five years and is renewable for five-year periods. On a number of occasions, the CPMP has requested post-marketing commitments as a condition of authorisation, and such commitments must be met within the timeframes stated in an Annex to the CPMP opinion. A pictorial presentation of the centralised procedure, including timeframes, is provided in Figure 4.2.

## European regulators and industry consultation

As highlighted above, European regulatory structures encourage, if not compel, regulatory agencies to engage in dialogue and to consult with industry both before and during the evaluation process. This has led some, if not all, of the national regulatory agencies to launch 'marketing campaigns' aimed at raising their profiles and at convincing industry of using their 'regulatory services'. Such marketing is connected with an agency's perceived need to persuade companies that it is open to dialogue and consultation both before and during evaluation.

For example, in 1994, in preparation for entry into the EU, the Swedish MPA employed an international consultancy firm to survey European industry's attitude, knowledge and awareness of the agency. The survey found that the MPA had 'an extremely good image among European companies and high credibility' (Burson Marsteller 1994). The industry was extremely positive about the MPA regarding approval time, competence and documentation. A second survey in 1995 found that European industry ranked the MPA as the second most favoured agency (behind the British MCA, which is widely regarded as the most 'promotional' regulatory agency in Europe). The results showed that 93 per cent of senior industry officials saw the agency as 'very willing' to enter into dialogue with companies, while the remaining 7 per cent felt that it was 'willing' (Burson Marsteller 1995).

The MPA's survey also asked industry officials to rank the

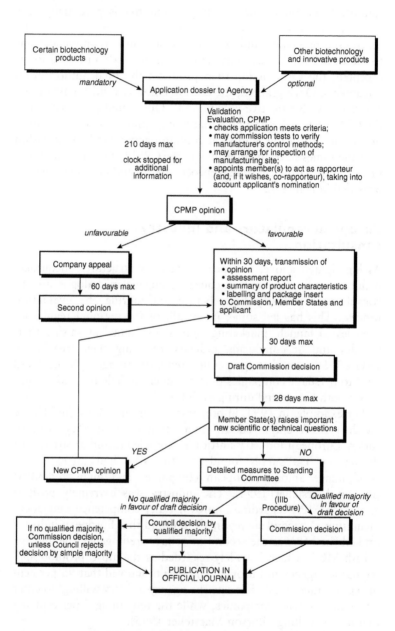

*Figure 4.2*    The EU's centralised procedure for marketing
authorisation of new drugs

criteria used for choosing a Reference Member State. The most common factors mentioned were (in descending order):

- speed of approval;
- experience and ability to negotiate in the EU;
- competence and quality of regulatory expertise;
- openness and willingness to co-operate with industry;
- clear communication;
- good approval history.

According to more than 90 per cent of the industry respondents, the MPA matched these criteria 'very well'. Industry felt that the MPA's strengths were: openness for dialogue and co-operation; the quality and speed of regulatory review; high quality assessment reports and reviewers; performance-oriented; pragmatic and flexible; and very open for pre-submission discussions. The consultants concluded their report by saying that the MPA had the potential to become 'the number one' regulatory agency in the EU because its strengths matched the criteria used when companies choose a Reference Member State (Burson Marsteller 1995). This telling conclusion indicates that the MPA's consultants had conceived of a successful regulatory agency as one which matches the wishes of the industry.

Like national drug regulatory agencies, the CPMP has been concerned to define its relations with companies, both to control the time spent on giving advice and to offset charges of involvement in the drug development process. The demand for scientific advice is growing, which suggests that it is important to industry, and that the industry is confident of success in seeking it. There were 78 requests for advice in the period 1995–8; 52 of these occurred in 1998, 43 of which were agreed to, including 16 oral consultations (EMEA 1999g).

Moves to clarify the issue of consultation have resulted in the CPMP publishing a 'standard operating procedure' on the subject. Accordingly, a company wanting advice must clearly identify the questions and issues to be addressed and the reasons why advice is being requested; and, in particular, 'why existing publications and guidelines cannot be used' (European Commission 1996a: 34). The CPMP decides whether to give advice on a case-by-case basis, and if it agrees to do so it normally appoints a member to provide the advice (ibid.). The giving of advice often involves complex multidisciplinary issues, and to restrict access to the CPMP itself, CPMP

Working Parties are often used for this process (EMEA 1996b; Anon 1996).[15] Recently, this aspect of CPMP work has been brought together under the Scientific Advice Review Group. The Group's aim is to present an integrated view with respect to quality, biotechnology, safety, efficacy and pharmacovigilance, drawing its membership from each of the CPMP Working Parties. To this end, it is charged with compiling a scientific advice database to ensure consistency over time and across therapeutic areas (EMEA 1999b).

In practice, companies often want to raise administrative/procedural questions as well as scientific ones, and to do this at an early stage in the development of innovative products. In the initial stages of the 'strong' European regulatory state, there was considerable uncertainty in industry circles over whether the EMEA would provide the same 'pre-submission' dialogue as companies had come to expect from some national authorities. According to the EMEA's director, official guidelines did not cover the subject of 'dialogue and advice' in a convincing way, possibly because they were 'written by authorities who were not accustomed to such dialogue' (Anon 1995d: 764). Reportedly, EMEA officials aim to make the agency *as approachable for companies as possible*. While technical advice is not given on a routine basis, advice is given for innovative products at an early stage of development (months or even years prior to submission), where there are no existing guidelines (Anon 1995d). However, according to the EMEA, the Agency's staff will not 'act as a consultant to pharmaceutical companies' or tell companies how to run clinical trials or conduct their research. In this way, the EMEA has sought to distinguish its approach from that of the FDA, where, according to the EMEA, 'companies seem to be losing responsibility' for their clinical studies. As Dower notes, the EMEA/CPMP believes its role lies in the checking of companies' data, not telling them what data to gather (Dower 1995). By 1999, around one hundred instances of advice had been provided by the CPMP (EMEA 1999b: Annex I).

## The role and selection of CPMP rapporteurs

One interesting aspect raised by the new authorisation arrangements is the changing role of the rapporteur before and after January 1995. First, however, it should be noted that the term 'rapporteur' was used to describe the Member State responsible for providing a first assessment in both the multi-state and concertation procedures. After January 1995, the terminology applies to the centralised procedure only, with the lead agency in the decentralised procedure referred to as the Reference Member State. The task of the rapporteur is to co-ordinate the evaluation of the application. Under the old concertation procedure, the appointed rapporteur was a Member State. As noted previously, CPMP members are now 'individual appointees', not representatives of Member States, and the CPMP appoints rapporteurs for applications submitted via the centralised procedure as 'individual' CPMP members. The EMEA must also take account of the competence of Member States' authorities and their ability to handle the work in a timely fashion. Officially, balancing rapporteurships across Member States is one way of improving the expertise available to national agencies, particularly the smaller ones, and there is anecdotal evidence to suggest that co-rapporteurships are sometimes awarded on this basis. According to the Commission, 'all [CPMP] members should have equal opportunities to play the role of rapporteur or co-rapporteur' and members are invited to express their preferences for upcoming rapporteurships (European Commission 1996a: 37).

Under the concertation procedure, a company could choose the Member State it wanted to act as rapporteur for its application. However, under the centralised procedure companies may merely express their preferences regarding rapporteurs. The CPMP is said to take these preferences into account, but there is no way of knowing if, and how, they do this. Fernand Sauer, the EMEA director, has described a principle of rotation in the following way:

> Under the system of rotation, the CPMP chairman tries initially to identify suitable candidates. One important factor in this is the distinct differences in willingness/ability that exists in delegations for being chosen as rapporteur/co-rapporteur. Some delegations have said they would be satisfied with only one rapporteurship/co-rapporteurship for the whole year ... at the other extreme, some delegations will take everything!
> (Anon 1996c: 178)

There has been a significant change in the distribution of rapporteurships since the start of the centralised procedure in 1995, though the UK and France retain leading positions and three delegations accounted for 24 of the first 60 possible appointments.[16] Of the 18 converted concertation marketing authorisation applications, the UK had 9 rapporteurships, France 3, Belgium and Italy 2 each and the Netherlands 1. Under the new system, the distribution of rapporteurs/co-rapporteurs for the 30 submitted marketing authorisation applications was as follows in early 1996: UK 9; France 8; Germany 7; Denmark, Ireland, Sweden 5; Austria, the Netherlands 4; Finland 3; Italy, Luxembourg, Portugal, Spain 2; and Greece 0 (Anon 1996c). As shown in Table 4.5, in 1998, for 32 active substances, the combined figures were: Sweden 10; France 9; Germany 8; the Netherlands 7; UK, Spain 5; Belgium, Ireland 4; Denmark, Finland, Italy 3; Austria, Portugal, Luxembourg 1; Greece 0 (EMEA 1999g).

There has also been a shift in the relative influence of the rapporteur and co-rapporteur in the assessment process. Originally, it was intended that they would be equal partners, but

Table 4.5  Centralised procedure: number of rapporteurs/ co-rapporteurs in different EU Member States, 1996 and 1998

| Member State | Early 1996* | 1998** |
|---|---|---|
| Austria | 4 | 1 |
| Belgium | n/a | 4 |
| Denmark | 5 | 3 |
| Finland | 3 | 3 |
| France | 8 | 9 |
| Germany | 7 | 8 |
| Greece | 0 | 0 |
| Ireland | 5 | 4 |
| Italy | 2 | 3 |
| Luxembourg | 2 | 1 |
| Netherlands | 4 | 7 |
| Portugal | 2 | 1 |
| Spain | 2 | 5 |
| Sweden | 5 | 10 |
| United Kingdom | 9 | 5 |

Notes:
* figures for 30 submitted marketing authorisation applications (Anon 1996a)
** figures for rapporteurships/co-rapporteurships (EMEA 1999g)

now the rapporteur is usually responsible for the assessment and the co-rapporteur merely validates the work. The 'European experts' used for assessments and to provide the CPMP with specific expertise are scientists put at the disposal of the EMEA by Member States (European Commission 1993b: Article 53). For example, all members of the UK CSM plus many other UK medical and scientific experts are on the list, and names have similarly been provided by all the other Member States. The total number of experts available to the CPMP numbers around 2,200 (EMEA 1999g). However, their identity remains hidden, largely at the behest of the UK which cites 'personal safety' reasons, despite the EMEA's stated commitment to greater 'openness' and the fact that data on UK experts is published in the UK. Reportedly, moves are afoot to publish this information, as well as CPMP members' interests. It is possible to request sight of the names, although the criteria used to decide whether to grant such requests are unclear (EMEA 1997b; EMEA 1999g).

The CPMP has also moved to clarify its own decision-making structure, adopting guidelines on how decisions are made. For decisions to be adopted, at least two-thirds of its members (i.e. at least 20) must be present, and the Committee is 'obliged to use its best endeavours to reach a scientific consensus'. If consensus cannot be reached, a majority opinion can be adopted, with abstentions unable to prevent adoption of an opinion by consensus or an absolute majority. If voting occurs, the result is published and divergent positions may be mentioned in the opinion (European Commission 1993a: Article 52; EMEA 1998b).

## Mutual recognition: making it work

In statistical terms, the history of mutual recognition prior to 1995 was one of failure. The multi-state procedure saw Member States raising objections to essentially every application submitted.[17] The crucial factor which increased the chances of successful mutual recognition was the introduction of binding arbitration into the operation of the CPMP. But, given the problems with the old multi-state procedure, success would also require a sea change in the attitude of Member States and their regulatory authorities towards mutual recognition. The present system has developed over many years and Member States have invested considerable political capital in it.

One criticism was that too much effort had gone into establishing the EMEA and the centralised procedure while ignoring unresolved problems with the decentralised procedure, which was expected to continue servicing the bulk of product applications. If industry confidence in and support for the new structures was undermined, the whole edifice of European authorisation could be called into question. Moreover, the largest authorities (except for Germany) rely on fees for their continued existence. In the run-up to its introduction in 1995, Member States expressed their intention to make the new mutual recognition procedure a success.

## Pharmacovigilance and harmonisation

So far our analysis of drug regulatory mechanisms has focused on pre-marketing requirements. The belief that drugs have already undergone rigorous comparisons of their usefulness and safety with other, older, products during clinical trials is commonplace (e.g. see Kerwin and Travis 1996; and the reply in Rawlins 1996). In reality, the basis of all approval systems, whether national or European, is that the assessment of safety and efficacy at the time of marketing is only provisional. Therefore, post-marketing surveillance, or pharmacovigilance as it is now termed, also forms an essential part of the (continuing) evaluation process. As we discussed in Chapter 1, a major reason for this is the fact that the pre-marketing safety database, consisting of pre-clinical and clinical data, is not sufficiently predictive to guarantee that a drug is safe for all patients at all times (Rawlins 1994).

Also, under the previous system of national licensing, the scale of exposure depended to a large extent on the speed with which national authorities conducted assessments. Although other factors influence a company's marketing strategy, differences in assessment times meant that marketing, and therefore patient exposure, tended to be staggered across the continent. Under the new 'efficiency regime', differences in the time that agencies take to assess products are decreasing under the impetus of EU-imposed timeframes and inter-agency competition. In particular, NASs are increasingly being approved via the centralised procedure, which permits the simultaneous marketing of products throughout the EU. Approval via mutual recognition, now compulsory for any 'non-centralised' product sold in more than one Member State, also serves to reduce the time to market in different Member

States. The trend is therefore towards simultaneous exposure of far larger populations in Europe than hitherto.

The lack of predictive value associated with pre-market testing, and the fact that products can now be sold throughout the EU much more easily than before underlie concern over pharmacovigilance standards in Europe. Hence, efforts to harmonise safety evaluation are directed not only at the pre-marketing stages of drug development, but also on the pharmacovigilance phase. However, reporting patterns between countries vary enormously. Thus, most commentators agree that better understanding of the reasons for this heterogeneity is needed before data from a larger population, such as the EU as a whole, can be analysed and interpreted as the sole basis for pharmacovigilance assessment

The basis of EU activity in this area derives from Article II of Directive 65/65/EEC, which states:

> The competent authorities of the Member States shall suspend or revoke an authorisation to place a proprietary medicinal product on the market where the product proves to be harmful in the normal conditions of use, or where its therapeutic efficacy is lacking when it is established that therapeutic results cannot be obtained with the proprietary product.
>
> (European Commission 1965: Article II)

Directive 75/319/EEC (European Commission 1975b) built on this framework by requiring Member States to take 'all appropriate measures to ensure that information relating to drug authorisations was communicated between them and, in particular, information relating to refusals, revocations, or product withdrawals', according to the head of the EMEA (Anon 1993j: 646).

In 1989 the first meeting was held of an expert group to advise the CPMP on matters related to ADRs and pharmacovigilance. Requirements for notifying Member States were strengthened somewhat in the same year, and an annual list of prohibited products has been published since 1992. The early 1990s also saw the publication by the CPMP of an overview of the subject, as well as documents on rapid alert systems, exchanging information, and a procedure on causality clarification (CPMP 1989; 1990; 1991a; 1991b).

As regards industry, formalised guidelines for reporting have now been introduced, including the submission of periodic safety updates. Companies must appoint a qualified person responsible for pharmacovigilance, who must ensure all suspected ADRs reported to the company are collected, evaluated and collated at a single point in the EU, and reports sent to the competent authorities. Requests for additional information must be answered fully and promptly, including information on sales or prescriptions. All suspected serious reactions from healthcare professionals must be reported to the competent authority within fifteen days and detailed records maintained of all other suspected ADRs reported to the company. These records have to be submitted to Member States on request, or at least every six months during the first two years after approval and once a year for the next three years, after which records and scientific evaluation are submitted every five years when applying for authorisation renewal or on request. Increasingly, to ensure compliance, companies are adopting measures to increase their control over the quality of data and to improve access. In other words, EU requirements are putting pressure on companies to improve their ADR systems.[18]

Member States continue to be responsible for national pharmacovigilance arrangements, which include reporting suspected ADRs immediately to the EMEA, and the company concerned within fifteen days of notification; and informing the EMEA and the company concerned whenever ADRs lead to the conclusion that a marketing authorisation should be amended, suspended or withdrawn. A product may be suspended without prior EU co-ordination on grounds of urgency, provided the EMEA is informed no later than the following working day. Under the centralised procedure, the CPMP can also take measures to ensure safe and effective use of medicinal products licensed by the EU, including any action required following emergency suspension of use of a product by a Member State.

Officially, the EMEA co-ordinates pharmacovigilance activities undertaken by Member States. Its functions in this area include informing Member States about suspected serious adverse reactions reported by other Member States; operating an electronic information network for rapid transmission of data between Member States; and collaborating with the World Health Organisation (WHO) on international pharmacovigilance. Nonetheless, despite plans to co-ordinate efforts on a European-wide basis, in practice individual Member States adopt different approaches when it comes to making decisions about potentially unsafe products already on the market, as does the CPMP on occasion.

It is worth noting that EU pharmacovigilance policy also inter-acts with public health policy in Member States, and even with the future of national agencies, as discussed in Chapters 5 and 6. For example, like other Member States, the UK is steadily moving towards linking surveillance with health outcome monitoring in a bid to reduce costs, and, in the UK case, also to reduce the arbi-trary rationing of new and untested therapies (Anon 1997i). The demand to exclude products with poor cost/efficacy ratios is likely to grow in all EU countries.

## The transposition of EU legislation into national law

Our discussion of the Europeanisation of medicines regulation would not be complete without some mention of how EU legisla-tive developments have affected national legal frameworks. European law takes precedence over domestic legislation in Member States, though some distinctively national regulations remain. For example, some very basic matters such as the defini-tion of a 'proprietary medicinal product' are not the same in British and EU law. EU law excludes surgical and dental materials, medical devices, products prepared in a pharmacy and homeo-pathic products. Also, the elaborate system of appeals afforded to manufacturers under the 1968 UK Medicines Act finds no place in the Europeanised procedures for medicines regulation. In this section, we consider only Sweden and the UK to illustrate the interaction between EU legislation and changes in national laws.

Most of the regulatory requirements contained in the three original EU Directives (65/65/EEC, 75/318/EEC and 75/319/EEC) were already covered by existing UK law: that is, the 1968 Medicines Act. Thus, implementation of these early 'framework' Directives mainly involved codification of various cumulative changes required to bring the UK fully into line with European obligations. Of particular importance are a number of Statutory Instruments enacted in 1993 and 1994. In 1993, new UK regula-tions designed to implement 75/318/EEC set out requirements regarding the data to be submitted with new drug applications, such as the inclusion of the summary of product characteristics, which superseded the specifically British data sheet.

The next year, UK legislation implemented all three EU frame-work Directives. This was explained in a British government document entitled *The Medicines for Human Use (Marketing Authorisations, Pharmacovigilance and Related Matters): Regulations 1994.* Apart from highlighting the terminological change from 'product licensing' to 'marketing authorisation', this also made UK legislation consistent with the EU obligations implied by the decentralised procedure for mutual recognition, the centralised procedure and pharmacovigilance (Anon 1994m). In particular, the MCA's obligation to recognise the arbitration procedure established under the decentralised procedure became enshrined in UK law, including the rights of national regulatory agencies from other Member States to request information on granting, varying, renewal or progress of marketing authorisation applications.[19]

Similar developments occurred in other Member States. The situation was slightly different in Sweden, which did not join the EU until January 1995. However, even there, medicines regulation had already been largely brought into line with EU requirements under 1994 agreements within the European Economic Area, which embraces the EU and the countries in the European Free Trade Area (EFTA) – of which Sweden was a member prior to membership of the EU. As with the UK, in Sweden Europeanisation of the legal framework for drug regulation concerned requirements of the decentralised procedure, mutual recognition, the centralised procedure and the mandatory inclusion of a summary of product characteristics for all marketing authorisation applications. Furthermore, it is no coincidence that the Swedish Medicinal Product Ordinance of 1993 specified drug product review times entirely consistent with those recommended by the European Commission, such as a maximum of 210 days for regulatory review of NASs.

Some aspects of the Europeanisation process affected Sweden specifically. For example, only drug approvals granted in Sweden after 1 January 1994 (that is, after the EEA agreements) could be used in the EU decentralised procedure. More significantly, the Swedish MPA was obliged to drop 'first choice' and 'second choice' classification of products. Previously, new products of equivalent effectiveness were classified by the agency as 'second choice' because of limited information about their adverse effects, while older, more established products were preferred for treatment ('first choice'). Such provisions can no longer be attached to a marketing authorisation in Sweden if there is no proven health risk. A statement in the MPA's 'information' publication to doctors suggests a degree of concern about this development (Anon 1994n).

## Conclusion

Medicines regulation in the EU is more complex than any national regulatory system. Drawing on Weber's concept of 'ideal type', Stone-Sweet and Sandholtz (1997) suggest that EU policy-making can be understood by reference to a continuum stretching between two ideal typical poles, namely 'intergovernmental politics' and 'supranational governance'. At its most simple, within the European regulatory state, the decentralised (mutual recognition) procedure approximates to 'intergovernmental politics' in which national regulators of Member States bargain with each other to produce common policies. On the other hand, the centralised procedure approximates to 'supranational governance' because it involves regulatory institutions centralised at the EU level which are capable of constraining the behaviour of all actors, including Member States in specific policy domains. It is clear from this model that when mutual recognition is not initially forthcoming, resulting in CPMP arbitration, then the nature of EU policy-making, in effect, moves along the continuum away from 'intergovernmental politics' towards 'supranational governance'.

We have characterised developments in the Europeanisation of medicines regulation since 1995 as a shift from a 'weak' to a 'strong' European regulatory state in the pharmaceuticals sector. That strength is, however, primarily in relation to national regulatory agencies. Mainly, power and authority has shifted from Member States to supranational bodies, rather than from industry to supranational bodies, though there are some instances of the latter. In fact, the 'strong' European regulatory state, which has been established, is largely the model of Europeanisation proposed by industry in the late 1980s, except that the key role of the CPMP has been retained.

The Europeanisation process involves pre-market and post-market aspects of drug evaluation, but the former is much more developed in terms of bureaucracy and formal procedures. The number of assessments which have achieved mutual recognition has dramatically increased since 1995. The evidence suggests that this cannot be explained by reference to purely technical and scientific matters. It is also important to appreciate that the development of procedures to harmonise pharmacovigilance across Europe is bound to affect the nature of the regulatory sciences involved. In the next chapter, we explore in more detail the interaction between the harmonisation of regulatory procedures and scientific expertise.

Chapter 5

# The politics of scientific expertise

As explained in Chapter 4, in January 1995 there were three key developments: CPMP opinions in both mutual recognition and concertation/centralised procedures became binding on Member States; the EMEA was established to administer the new procedures, with expert advice from the CPMP; and strict timetables for product assessment were introduced. These changes signalled the latest and most important stage in the introduction of an 'efficiency regime' for pharmaceuticals in Europe. In January 1998, the parallel national application route disappeared, making it no longer possible to market a drug in more than one EU country via the national licensing authorities, apart from generics and herbal products (European Commission 1997).

In this chapter, we focus on how the new EU regulatory regime is attempting to *make* harmonisation a success through the imposition of political, bureaucratic and institutional change. In particular, we examine the implications of this for the regulatory process, especially European scientific expertise, national regulatory agencies and national scientific advisory committees. Most attention is given to harmonisation under the decentralised procedure because that is where the most significant issues of mutual recognition arise, but we also discuss these issues with reference to the centralised procedure and European post-marketing surveillance (pharmacovigilance). This is of most relevance to medicines safety and efficacy considerations rather than medicinal quality, because the latter tends to generate less (international) scientific dispute.

## The background of failure for the multi-state procedure

In Chapter 4, we described the historical and legislative process by which new regulatory structures, in the form of mutual recognition and the concertation/centralised procedures, have steadily transformed the regulatory environment for pharmaceuticals in Europe. In quantitative terms, however, the history of EU mutual recognition, in particular, is one of failure. Prior to 1995, the multi-state procedure saw Member States raising objections to all but one of the applications submitted. Furthermore, data from the European Commission show that manufacturers rarely used the multi-state procedure, preferring instead to use parallel national applications. This was particularly true for the larger companies, who had the least to gain in terms of 'economies of scale', because they generally have the resources available locally to process national applications.

Our research shows that when companies did use the multi-state procedure, it was often to gain experience of the system using unimportant products or for 'mopping up' – a term used to describe situations where multi-state approval is sought in smaller markets after the most important authorisations have been obtained via national applications. As a regulatory affairs director at a leading Swedish company put it:

> We have used it [multi-state procedure] but we were reluctant. We looked at the outcome of that procedure and it was not good at all. We said we can try to use it just to get acquainted with the process on some products we didn't consider that important, in countries [markets] that were not that important.[1]

This illustrates how the perceived risks of the multi-state procedure, compared with the company's experience of national applications, induced the company to 'play safe' by using the procedure mainly for less important products. However, where those perceived risks could be alleviated, companies were enticed to use the procedure for more significant products, such as NASs. For example, this same company had a good personal toxicology contact at the Dutch regulatory authorities, and this helped the company develop the confidence to use the procedure with the Dutch regulators acting as rapporteur. Such findings confirm the role of interpersonal networking within the multi-state procedure noted in previous research (Abraham and Charlton 1995).

## The new regime and the 'virtual' Euro-agency

In addition to the European Commission, two important EU organisations specifically concerned with harmonising regulatory science in the pharmaceutical sector are the EMEA (since January 1995) and the more long-standing CPMP. As described in Chapter 4, the CPMP becomes involved in the decentralised procedure only if the Concerned Member States do not mutually recognise the assessment of the Reference Member State, in which case the company's application goes to arbitration. The CPMP then comes to an opinion at arbitration and the Commission drafts a decision based on that opinion, which is ratified by a Standing Committee of non-scientific representatives of Member States (by qualified majority vote). If the draft decision is not supported by a qualified majority of the Standing Committee, then it is referred to the Council of Ministers. Once agreement is reached by either the Standing Committee or the Council of Ministers, it becomes a Commission or Council decision. Member States then translate that decision into the provision of a Europeanised 'national' licence (see Figure 4.1). By contrast, the CPMP is necessarily involved in the centralised procedure and drives a regulatory process culminating in the authorisation (or not) of an EU licence by the Commission or the Council. While Member States can raise important scientific objections to the rapporteur's assessment, they do so in the context of a Europeanised procedure in which the CPMP are already involved (see Figure 4.2). Thus, mutual recognition plays a much less significant role than in the decentralised procedure. Throughout both procedures, the EMEA acts as the CPMP's scientific secretariat.

Officially, the Standing Committee is not supposed to intervene in 'scientific' matters. Nevertheless, consensus at the CPMP does not automatically result in harmonisation, because of the possibility of intervention by Member States via the Standing Committee. This is evident from cases in which the Standing Committee was divided over the availability of Schering AG's multiple sclerosis therapy, Betaferon (beta-interferon) and Rhone-Poulenc Rorer's anti-cancer agent, Taxotere (docetaxel), both recommended for approval by the CPMP. Sweden wanted to avoid excessive prescribing restrictions on both medicines, but because of cost considerations the British health authorities issued guidelines

restricting prescriptions for them to specialists, while in Germany
BfArM permitted Betaferon to be advertised in publications sent
to all doctors, not just specialist clinicians (Anon 1996b).

The EMEA has a Management Board consisting of two representatives from each Member State, two from the Commission
and two from the European Parliament. In this respect, it may be
seen as a typically European arrangement in which the executive
and legislative responsibilities are fused into a co-operative, rather
than competitive, relationship regarding the bureaucracy. The
absence of legislative–executive competition, as occurs between
Congress and the Administration in the US, minimises rigorous
legislative and procedural controls on the EMEA. Consequently,
the EMEA enjoys considerable independence in interpreting and
implementing regulatory policy. While the EMEA's Management
Board is obliged to forward an annual report on its activities and
a programme of work for the forthcoming year to Member States,
the Commission and the European Parliament, it seems likely that
EU regulators will be able to make trade-offs and compromises
without presenting public justification to a European
Parliamentary Committee, in the way that US regulators in the
FDA have been required to defend their decisions before
Congressional Committees. Among the main official objectives of
EMEA are to:

- protect and promote public health by providing safe and
  effective medicines; give patients quick access to new innovative therapy;
- facilitate the free movement of pharmaceutical products
  throughout the EU; harmonise scientific requirements to
  optimise pharmaceutical research worldwide;
- provide Member States and EU institutions with the best
  possible scientific advice on quality, safety and efficacy of
  medicines;
- establish a multinational scientific expertise through the
  mobilisation of existing national resources in order to
  achieve a single evaluation via a centralised or decentralised
  marketing authorisation;
- organise speedy, transparent and efficient procedures for
  the authorisation, surveillance and withdrawal of products
  in the EU.

(EMEA 1996a: 9)

All Member States contribute to the EMEA's operations because all scientific assessment activity for which the EMEA is responsible (e.g. in the centralised procedure) is actually conducted by national assessors on a fee-basis, with the EMEA providing administrative and IT services for meetings of the CPMP and associated experts. This approach is consistent with a long-standing reluctance of European countries to build up substantial central resources of regulatory scientific expertise, and with a concern in those countries to minimise administrative costs (Brickman et al. 1985: 160, 303). In this sense the EMEA is a *virtual regulatory agency*. As a senior member of the German regulatory authority, BfArM, described it: 'EMEA is a funny construction because in part it is a complete European institution but it is also a virtual institution because to a certain degree every [national] agency is part of EMEA through the CPMP and other channels.'[2]

This is because the expertise of the CPMP has been built on the national resources of Member States. Both the centralised and decentralised procedures are based on the use of such national resources. For example, the 'Euro-experts' used for assessments of applications in the centralised procedure are, in effect, scientists put at the disposal of the EMEA by Member States (as required by Article 53 of Council Regulation (EC) No. 2309/93).

## The CPMP: representing politics as science

The exclusion of all but 'expert scientists' from CPMP deliberations is justified officially on the grounds that the Committee's decision-making is confined to scientific matters that demand members with the requisite technical knowledge. As previously noted, a similar official rationale underpins the division of responsibilities between the 'scientific' CPMP and the 'political' Standing Committee. As part of the Commission's strategy to promote harmonisation, this rationale has been further applied to the CPMP. Prior to 1995, membership of the CPMP was on a 'representational' basis – one member per Member State. However, under the new regulatory regime members are said to be appointed on an 'individual basis', described as reflecting scientific competence. In addition, since January 1995, the EMEA and the CPMP have appointed rapporteurs for applications submitted via the centralised procedure as 'individual' CPMP members rather than as representatives of Member States, as occurred before 1995. In principle, these arrangements allow the rapporteur to construct a drug product assessment team using expertise from different national regulatory agencies with, say, the safety section of the application being assessed by scientists at the MCA and the efficacy section being assessed by scientists at BfArM. Some observers claim that 'individual' membership encourages CPMP members to be more independent, compared to when they were representatives of a Member State. On this argument, under the old arrangement, members would automatically support the view of their national agency at meetings rather than consider issues 'objectively'. For example, according to the Head of the EMEA's Human Medicines Unit, these changes have made the CPMP more 'scientific': 'It was formerly membership for a member state, and now it's membership for personal reasons and abilities and, therefore, the discussions have changed very much, reaching into scientific details.'[3]

The difficulties that regulators had in mutually recognising other Member States' assessments prior to 1995 are of some relevance here to the interaction between science and politics in EU drug regulation. Some of our informants suggested that the differences between Member States' supposedly technical assessments were not solely scientific. Regarding the reasons for lack of mutual recognition, a highly experienced official at the Swedish regulatory authority, the MPA, commented: 'My experience so far is that there's a lot more to it than science. Yes. It's a lot more than science. ... there are national traditions ... or medical practice.'[4]

The thinking behind amplifying the 'scientific status' of the CPMP was to reduce the role of such national differences within the CPMP on the assumption that regulatory science is 'universalistic' (Merton 1942). In particular, the new selection criteria for members were intended to counter concerns that CPMP members were compelled to adopt the view of their national authority when participating in CPMP discussions, thus submerging their 'scientific' judgement in favour of national political interests (Anon 1996c).

This scientistic perspective on CPMP decision-making was clearly articulated by the Head of the EMEA's Human Medicines Unit, who described it as follows:

> You have a discussion until you reach a compromise, and all discussions have led to consensus, which means it's not voting, me against you, west against east, or north against south, but it's really listening to arguments and trying to come to an

understanding. This can only be done on a scientific rationale. If you rely on your government, on national background, it's not going to work.[5]

Yet, in reality, detaching politics from science in European medicines regulation has proved much more difficult. An examination of regulatory structures after 1995 shows that there remained 'representational' and 'political' elements. For example, since 1995 there have been two members per Member State, instead of one, and most Member States continued to be 'represented' by the top officials from their national agencies. Indeed, the membership of the 'old' and 'new' CPMP remained largely unchanged, including the chair and vice-chair. Furthermore, under the centralised procedure, assessments invariably have been conducted by the national agencies to which the appointed rapporteur belongs. Our evidence suggests that product assessments using expertise from different national agencies are yet to happen to any degree, although this could change over time.[6] In fact, the extent to which rapporteurs are selected according to individual scientific expertise is compromised, because EMEA sources told us that awarding 'too many' rapporteurships to the same country would not make 'good politics'.[7] Officially, 'the preference of the applicant is not followed if an imbalance in the rapporteurships of interested members would be the consequence' and applicants are advised to specify several preferences 'from different delegations' to increase the likelihood that their choice is followed (European Commission 1996a: 37).

Consequently, national differences in medical outlook may manifest themselves at the European level through the CPMP because the Committee's membership have the dual role of 'technical scientist' and 'national bureaucrat'. In some cases the bureaucratic/political role may be more significant, and this may explain why a harmonisation process based on universalistic assumptions about science has proved inadequate. Thus, one argument against expecting much change is that CPMP members still have to work in their 'own' agencies, and are therefore not 'free agents' but subject to the same bureaucratic and political constraints as before. As one MPA scientist revealed:

There are actually very few pure technical people [on the CPMP]. I don't know how the individual members, all of them, how they work nationally. Of course, we are members of the CPMP and shouldn't take too much influence of what our own [national] agency believes. But, of course, our views are reflected by the views of our organisation ... It's not possible [to remove national influences] because you're working in the agency and you rely on the expertise and you cannot always be on top of every issue yourself. You gather information from a lot of people, from outside and inside, and you are influenced to a large extent by the internal organisation.[8]

This view was confirmed by a senior German regulator at BfArM, who commented:

The CPMP itself is not the body to do any science. There is a big difference between the theory that this is a commission of people with big scientific backgrounds and the reality that this is a collection of European administrators ... CPMP members are all administrators in national authorities and what they are discussing, everything the CPMP is doing, will have effects on their own area of responsibility at home, so they have to take this into consideration ... This is not pure science usually. Take oral contraceptives, for example. What is worse, to prevent a certain amount of thrombotic events, but get so many more women pregnant that didn't want to be that there are more abortions?[9]

Similarly, another Swedish regulator explained the fundamental difficulty in making clear-cut divisions between science and politics in medicines regulation because the acceptability of risk-benefit ratios is neither universalistic nor scientistic:

How much value you put in a particular cancer finding in one rat study versus the relative efficacy of the drug in treating an illness is not an easy judgement. Some people say, yes, this is an acceptable finding, but still approve the drug. Some people will say no. It's difficult to know which one is right. No-one knows.[10]

The implication of this analysis is that the similarity in outlook among toxicologists and clinicians, which may have characterised the relatively small and homogeneous research communities of individual European Member States, needs to undergo reformulation into an 'epistemic community' at the European level in order for the harmonisation of EU medicines regulation to progress (Haas 1992). Moreover, that reformulation necessarily involves political and bureaucratic changes, some of which we discuss below, despite the official representations of the process as one of technical consensus.

## Informality, efficiency and transparency

As previously noted, the EMEA aims to provide speedy, transparent and efficient procedures for marketing authorisations that give patients quick access to new therapies in the EU. There is an implicit assumption that these goals cannot, and do not, conflict. However, too often governments and other political organisations interpret 'speed' and 'efficiency' as synonymous with minimal consultation. A frequent casualty of such an approach is transparency.

It is clear from Figure 4.1 that if Member States go to arbitration then the decentralised procedure is much more protracted. As noted in Chapter 4, in the interests of expediency, the UK, Germany and France agreed to be 'good Europeans' at an informal meeting immediately prior to the start of the new system. By this informal channel they agreed to restrict arbitration to four areas, namely indications, contra-indications/warnings, dosage, and shelf-life; and agreed *in advance* to automatic mutual recognition of the rest of the drug product application that had no bearing on these four areas (Dower 1995).

Despite these efforts, by late 1995 doubts about mutual recognition surfaced in public when one senior German regulator described the decentralised procedure as being 'in chaos' (Anon 1995e). To counteract such reports and boost industry's confidence, the heads of national regulatory agencies met in the Netherlands in early 1996 to review the EU drug licensing systems. The meeting stressed the importance of national agencies, describing them as the 'backbone of the European licensing system'. It also confirmed that only 'issues of risk to public health' would be considered during days 60 to 90 of the procedure and insisted that, despite misconceptions about the new system, experience to date had been satisfactory. In a key development, the agency heads also committed themselves to 'jointly oversee the execution of the mutual recognition procedure' (Heads of Medicines Agency 1996).

This meeting signalled the existence of the Mutual Recognition Facilitation Group (MRFG), an informal grouping of regulatory authority directors or senior officials which meets under the unofficial auspices of the CPMP. Apparently its principal function is to facilitate the successful operation of the decentralised procedure and is a direct outcome of the failure of mutual recognition under the multi-state procedure and doubts about the viability of its successor, the decentralised procedure. However, it is not an official body and is not mentioned in any Directive or Regulation.

According to a senior BfArM official, the MRFG is not meant to solve any problems itself, but to agree on ways and means to do so. In other words, it is supposed to improve mutual recognition, rather than provide a forum for the resolution of scientific issues.[11]

Because its membership closely matches that of the CPMP, the MRFG meets in London as an adjunct to the monthly CPMP meeting. In addition, there is also the Heads of National Regulatory Authorities Group, another important 'unofficial' forum, in the sense that it does not exist in any Directive or other legislative document. It also facilitates discussion of issues connected with mutual recognition applications and European medicines harmonisation in general.

Considerable anecdotal evidence collected in the course of our research demonstrates the informality of many decisions and the importance of informal contacts for dispute resolution within the mutual recognition procedure. As one senior regulator at the EMEA told us:

> I think it's fair to state that it was believed that it [mutual recognition] could be run from home, by telephone, letters and faxes and e-mail. But apparently the discussions from person to person and in the group are very important to reach a consensus in mutual recognition, and this [the MRFG] is where we offer a platform for the Member States to act and react on.[12]

Asked if the MRFG had in fact been 'bolted-on' in ad hoc fashion once problems were recognised, a senior UK regulator described its formation in the following terms:

> It was bolted on, I think. People recognised that we had to do something to make mutual recognition work. It hadn't worked

under the old multi-state procedure and something had got to be done … [Its function is] to promote a common understanding and agreement on standards and approaches and procedures. And also a sort of broad common understanding of the kinds of issues on which things will be blocked, and the kinds of issues on which we will agree to differ, but perhaps let things go through.[13]

Because of its make-up and unofficial status, it is difficult to determine exactly where the work of the CPMP ends and that of the MRFG begins. In formal terms, the CPMP's competence extends to the assessment of centralised procedures, arbitration of mutual recognition disputes, and pharmacovigilance matters. But both regulators and industry speak of the need to avoid disputes going to CPMP arbitration. One way to view the MRFG's function is as an attempt to reduce the number of 'official' arbitration cases. Ironing out relatively minor problems and disagreements through personal contact at CPMP meetings avoids expensive, time-consuming, and potentially embarrassing arbitration procedures. However, little is known about the day-to-day operation of the MRFG, since it operates behind doors which are even more closed than those of the CPMP. Recently, MRFG membership has expanded to include more individuals from each national agency and the EMEA has begun to be more open about the existence of the MRFG. For example, it now issues a (brief) press release after meetings, along with other information about the MRFG; and members now include the fact that they are members in their personal biographies (EMEA 1999d; MRFG 1999).

Alongside the MRFG there have been a number of informal meetings arranged by national regulatory agencies for their scientific assessors, who actually evaluate applications, rather than the senior agency officials. Like the MRFG, the principal impetus for these meetings comes from the decentralised system. However, the most important element of these meetings is 'networking', not scientific discussion. As one senior regulator explained, speed and 'efficiency' are the motivating factors:

[The meetings] all have one very big main purpose and a small secondary purpose. The small secondary purpose is what you just mentioned [scientific discussion]. By far the more important purpose is just to give the opportunity for assessors to meet their opposite numbers. There is a possibility to get a personal relationship, to know what the other guy looks like. The science which is discussed ... is very nice, but is really not the most important part. It is our experience that collaboration between the various agencies is usually limited by the fact that there is a certain official contact level. Each agency has contact points to other agencies but these contact points are rather remote to the experts, and if every information goes via the contact points a lot of things are delayed and lost and it's not so good. We all want to encourage our assessors, if they are reading an assessment report and they don't understand anything, that they don't initiate a big bureaucratic procedure but instead ... pick up the phone, call the other guy and say look, I can't understand this, what did you think when you wrote this, and this is difficult to achieve when people don't know one another. So, for this sociological knowledge, at regular intervals for various [therapeutic] areas, meetings are arranged that assessors are invited to.[14]

Efforts to improve both the image and operation of the post-1995 mutual recognition procedure have extended beyond the regulators. In March 1996 the European Commission hosted a liaison meeting between Member States and industry representatives to discuss the operation of the procedure, at which it presented an upbeat account of usage and outcomes, and such meetings have occurred on a regular basis subsequently. At the meeting, various measures to encourage industry's participation were agreed. Industry representatives, for their part, expressed satisfaction 'at the frank and forthright discussion which had taken place, and commended the many practical improvements introduced' which would further enhance the procedure (European Commission 1996b).

Evidently, the determination to make mutual recognition successful has led to a proliferation of informality in European drug regulatory structures. Our analysis also shows how the development of a Europeanised model of regulation is based on the flexible British style in which policy and regulatory assessments are constructed through close, informal contacts, in preference to the traditionally more formalised approaches of Germany and the US (Brickman et al. 1985: 53, 247). Such informality may produce more rapid harmonisation, but it does raise important questions about transparency and accountability, not to mention the potential for industrial capture and social closure. Not only does the MRFG operate behind closed doors, as does the CPMP, but little is known about its activities. The EMEA provides brief press releases about CPMP meetings regarding drug products within the *centralised* procedure, and the heads of national regulatory agencies post brief minutes of MRFG meetings on their websites. Similar comments may be made about the increasingly informal meetings and discussions between the scientific assessors.

There has been more, and faster, mutual recognition under the decentralised procedure than under the multi-state procedure. This is being driven primarily by *bureaucratic and political means* and less by the open sharing and advancement of scientific understanding about the quality, safety and effectiveness of new drugs among the wider medical and public health community outside the regulator–industry network. These findings fundamentally challenge the official representation of European drug regulation as a scientific process, especially if one attaches any importance to the Mertonian ideal of open communication of knowledge across the 'scientific community'.

## The internal market and scientific peer review

The system of mutual recognition means that Concerned Member States review the Reference Member State's scientific assessment of the drug product application. Arguably, therefore, European mutual recognition procedures have extended scientific peer review in drug regulation. This is often cited as one way in which the decentralised procedure has raised the scientific quality of assessments. As one senior scientist at BfArM put it:

You can only survive the [European] system if what you are doing is scientifically sound. If you are doing anybody [i.e. a company] a favour, this might work on a purely national basis, but the moment you go into the European arena, you will have to explain this to others [the Concerned Member States] and this will be very difficult. ... This is not a move in the direction of making it easier for industry, in some respects it's even the opposite, but in some respects it's on a better, higher level now.[15]

On the other hand, it needs to be appreciated that most national regulatory agencies in the EU are almost entirely dependent on the fees which companies pay them to undertake regulatory assessments. The exception is BfArM in Germany, which is only dependent on industry fees for 40 per cent of its revenue. The most financially significant fees for national agencies within the European regulatory systems are generated by Reference Member State or rapporteur status, because they involve the production of the initial regulatory assessment. Such status is of additional importance to the regulatory institutions because it represents much more interesting and challenging scientific work than the 'checking' role that comes with Concerned Member State status. Consequently, by maximising its Reference Member State or rapporteur work, a national regulatory authority increases the likelihood of keeping and attracting good-quality scientists. All these factors have been magnified since January 1998, when parallel national applications disappeared and the European procedures increasingly came to dominate the regulatory workloads of the national agencies.

In effect, there exists an internal market in which national regulatory agencies compete with each other for regulatory business from industry, especially the most lucrative Reference Member State status. Representatives from industry told us consistently that they look for regulatory agencies who provide rapid assessments which lead to successful marketing authorisation because they are robust enough in quality to withstand the scrutiny of Concerned Member States.[16] Furthermore, industry demands for fast approval of new drugs are reflected in the strict timetable laid down by the Commission for decentralised and centralised applications. While the timetable is not legally enforceable, because Member States now compete for regulatory business from an industry that wants fast approvals they are under considerable pressure to conform.

In fact, such inter-agency competition has led the MCA to 'sell themselves' as the fastest in reviewing and approving drugs in the EU. Consequently, they are promoting themselves as being able to conduct regulatory assessments in less than the requisite 210 days. We found that the MCA were indeed popular among our industry sources. One praised them for 'wanting to license medicines, whereas with some authorities you get the feeling that they want to keep medicines off the market as much as possible'.[17] A regulatory affairs manager in a large UK company favoured the MCA because 'they understand the industry pressures, they know they have to bid for these applications to get them, they have to perform'.[18]

While MCA regulators insist that rapid assessment does not entail lower quality because of the need to satisfy the peer review by Concerned Member States,[19] many other regulators we interviewed were not convinced. For example, one Swedish scientist at the MPA argued that the new European procedures, especially the rapid timetables for mutual recognition, were *eroding peer review*, rather than enhancing it, by discouraging Concerned Member States to conduct their own independent assessments:

> Previously each drug was assessed in many countries, which of course was a waste of resources in one way, but you got second and third opinions on the same thing, which sometimes is not so bad ... and that type of safety check isn't there any more.[20]

As the selection of rapporteurs under the centralised procedure is made by the EMEA and CPMP, rather than by the applicants, the competition for rapporteurships among the national agencies has a rather different dynamic. Prior to 1995, under the concertation procedure, companies could choose the rapporteur. Not surprisingly, industry wanted to continue this arrangement in the centralised procedure, and industry associations lobbied intensively for the 'right to choose' to be kept. Instead, the EMEA/CPMP offered a compromise in which companies can tell the CPMP who they want to act as rapporteur. As noted in Chapter 4, this has made a difference (see Table 4.5). For example, at the end of the concertation procedure, the UK had half of all the rapporteurships, but by 1996 this had fallen to less than a third (Anon 1996b).[21] This suggests that the popularity of the MCA with industry in the regulators' 'market' has been modulated by the intervention of the EMEA. Hence, the national regulatory agency seeking rapporteurships must also persuade the EMEA that it has the best expertise for the job in addition to being popular with industry. Even then, an agency may be unsuccessful because of the Commission's 'political egalitarian' principle that all members should have equal opportunities to play the role of rapporteur.[22]

Under the centralised procedure the EMEA and the CPMP are always involved. By contrast, under the decentralised procedure the EMEA and the CPMP may not become involved, allowing all the revenue for regulatory work to flow to the national agency. Consequently, the competition between national agencies for rapporteurships under the centralised procedure is further dampened by the fact that the fees for them is much less than for Reference Member State status under the decentralised procedure. Moreover, the failure of mutual recognition would mean that the future of the national agencies could not be guaranteed, at least not at existing staffing levels. While all assessments within the mutual recognition procedure are conducted by national authorities, because companies are free to choose which authority they use for the initial assessment those agencies that are 'most efficient' and provide the 'best service' to industry can win more work than others. Indeed, the extent of this competition extends beyond what was presumably intended by the Commission, because it raises the possibility of national agencies seeking to persuade companies to take the decentralised, rather than the centralised, procedure for NASs. According to some German regulators, the principal fee-based agencies (such as Sweden and the UK) refuse to advise companies to use the centralised procedure because of the financial penalties they suffer if a company chooses that route.[23] As one senior BfArM official commented:

> If you talk to these agencies, or companies who have talked to them, you will hear that there is not one single case where they have given the advice to use the centralised system, even if it is to the disadvantage of the applicant.[24]

A regulatory affairs manager working for a company in Germany articulated the problem as follows:

> There is a down side [to inter-agency competition for fees]. This is that as soon as the regulators need a certain income, the money has to really flow in, and if their decision to fight for a product to get the application is based on the calculation of money and not anything else, it would be a disaster, and that has started already with the MCA. And other authorities are fighting for the decentralised mutual recognition procedure in cases where the centralised procedure would be more feasible, just because of the money.[25]

We have no documentary evidence to support these criticisms of some national regulatory authorities, so they should be viewed with some scepticism. Nevertheless, these criticisms were made by a number of our German sources at BfArM. It is notable that all of these criticisms emanated from Germany, where the regulatory agency is much less dependent on industry fees.

## The viability of national agencies

Despite the establishment of the EMEA and the new procedures involving *binding* 'scientific' opinions at the European level, national regulatory agencies are fundamental to EU medicines licensing, especially the mutual recognition procedure. When the Heads of Member States' regulatory agencies met in the Netherlands in early 1996 to review the EU drug licensing system, they emphasised that the national agencies were the 'backbone of the European licensing system' and reiterated the Member States' intention to 'jointly oversee the execution of the mutual recognition procedure' (Heads of Medicines Agency 1996). This *nationally*-grounded perspective on European medicines regulation was confirmed by the MPA's Head of Regulatory Administration in Sweden, who told us that he objected to the term 'decentralised' for the mutual recognition procedure because he viewed it as a 'trans*national*' process *without* delegation of responsibility from a central European body.[26]

It is these *national interests* that are also motivating the national agencies to make mutual recognition work without going to arbitration in the decentralised procedure. There are two main reasons for this. First, arbitration threatens to undermine a national agency's credibility both with industry and other regulatory agencies. If an agency approves a product which ends up being rejected in arbitration, then this sends a signal that that agency has misread or ignored the views of other Member States, and that it may be lacking in scientific and/or negotiating 'know-how'. And second, if Member States consistently fail to mutually recognise each other's assessments, the Commission and the EMEA are more likely to argue for centralisation. Such centralisation might move towards a European regulatory agency, similar to the FDA, with increasing independence from Member States. Developments of that kind would shift regulatory control and work away from the Member States to the EMEA and the CPMP with the consequent reduction in income for the national regulatory agencies. Hence, there is a convergence of interests between the industry and the national regulatory agencies to approve product applications quickly by mutual recognition.

There was general agreement among our respondents in government and industry that the British, Dutch, French, German and Swedish regulatory agencies were the five most experienced and competent in Europe. Many believe that, perhaps within the next decade, these will be the only five national agencies with the capacity to conduct full product assessments. This is based on the observation that the overwhelming majority of mutual recognition applications are currently undertaken by these five national agencies, and that this concentration of regulatory work is likely to increase because of inter-agency competition. Moreover, one German regulatory official claimed that some national agencies are already unable to assess applications properly under the centralised procedure.[27] On this view, the medium or long-term prognosis for some national agencies in the EU is that they will withdraw from 'first line' drug product assessment, but maintain an administrative capability in order to collect and analyse pharmacovigilance data for drugs already on the market. 'Local' pharmacovigilance capability is necessary in order to comply with EU requirements and, arguably, for domestic political reasons also.

## The viability of national scientific advisory committees

Historically, public confidence in the safety and efficacy of medicines rests, in part, on the national expert science advisory committee system. This is especially true in the UK, where the expert advisory system for medicines is more influential than any other Member State. Indeed, as we outlined in Chapter 3, in the UK the drug regulatory edifice is founded largely on using 'independent' external experts to judge the safety and efficacy of products.

There are two basic models of national advisory committees which may be seen as extremes on a continuum. At one extreme, the executive and advisory committee structures are essentially one and the same thing, as in the Netherlands. At the other, the function of advisory committees is *purely* advisory and the executive power of decision-making rests entirely with the national agency, as occurs in Germany. The British and Swedish committee systems lie between these two extremes. In the UK, the committee system is essentially advisory, but evidently grants considerable power to its principal expert advisory committee, the CSM, because the Committee's advice is nearly always accepted by the MCA. The Swedish model grants sole right of decision-making to the Director General of the MPA, although the agency seldom decides against the advice of its expert committee, the BOD. However, unlike the British model, the Director General occupies the pivotal position of being both Head of the MPA and Chairperson of the BOD – a situation which may encourage the BOD to align itself more readily with the will of the agency. As regards the situation in Germany, the BfArM is officially required to seek the advice of its expert committee, Kommission A, but a senior regulatory official told us that the German regulatory authority ignores the views of the committee if they conflict with those of BfArM.[28]

Our research suggests that the Europeanisation of medicines regulation is likely to diminish, if not marginalise or abolish, the role of national expert advisory committees of whatever variety. This is because the EU timeframes, which commit national agencies to complete assessments rapidly, place tremendous strain on advisory committees composed of 'outside' experts. Furthermore, certain features of the European licensing system, especially the mutual recognition procedure, suggest a more limited role for such committees. For example, one MCA official implied that the maintenance of the CSM's current role is dependent on the agency's success in securing Reference Member State status:

> While we are a leading Reference Member State, and at the moment we are *the* leading Reference Member State, the CSM has its usual role, except that, to keep to the timescale, it's got a smaller core membership who meet more often.[29]

This follows from the fact that the CSM's role is reduced when the UK is a Concerned Member State in the mutual recognition procedure. As this MCA official explained:

> When we are a Concerned Member State, it's obviously a reduced role. We will accept the Reference Member State's authorisation unless there is a major scientific objection. In

some instances we may want to consult the CSM. The CSM has been used to going through and making sure that every-thing is exactly as they would want it. Clearly, they will have a slightly different remit when we are a Concerned Member State ... [because then] the RMS has done the evaluation, we in the MCA have reviewed it, but there may be one issue we would like the CSM to address, rather than give the CSM the full dossier.[30]

In fact, a senior clinical assessor at the MCA told us that, when the agency is a Concerned Member State, it 'no longer takes all the advice of the CSM' because, under the European procedures, the Concerned Member State 'can only raise major objections on the grounds of public health'.[31] This admission demonstrates some of the practical implications of the rule which restricts arbitration to the four criteria: indications; contraindications/warnings; dosage; and shelf-life.

Similarly, according to the MPA, because of the imposition of timescales it is not possible for the Swedish BOD to examine all applications under the centralised procedure, which previously would have been reviewed by the Board. As one senior MPA official told us, the BOD will be 'more informed, rather than involved'.[32] Regarding the mutual recognition procedure, he surmised: 'With the decentralised procedure in full operation [from January 1998 when parallel national applications disappeared], the Board, as it works now, will become redundant. We'll have to find other means of bringing those external specialists into our work.'[33]

Indeed, a clinical expert member of the BOD admitted fatalisti-cally: 'To be frank, my feeling is that we [the BOD] will, on the whole, be less important and what our role will be in the new system is quite difficult to say.'[34]

Thus, if the MPA wants to continue expert advisory committee participation in regulatory decisions, there is a trade-off between complying with EU rules and maintaining effective links with the BOD. When asked how 'outside' experts could remain involved in MPA assessment work within the EU framework, a senior assessor at the agency replied:

What we have discussed is to bring them [expert advisors] in earlier in the evaluation process and not, as in the present situ-ation, bring all the specialists together to look at a number of applications, but rather bring in a few specialists within that therapeutic area and maybe have one or two clinical pharmacologists with a broader view of drug evaluation. Also bring them in more often into our project groups who work with the evaluations.[35]

This implies that Europeanisation of medicines regulation is blurring the conventional division between 'internal' scientific assessors and 'outside' independent experts in at least one Member State. These changes also suggest increased reliance on specialists, rather than on generalists, which may detract from the experts' independence because of over-identification with the drug products under review. It has been argued that, in the US, such over-identification can lead to problems of conflicts of interest, because of the greater likelihood of drawing on experts who have built their careers on developing drugs similar to the one being evaluated (Abraham and Sheppard 1996).

Indeed, on at least one occasion the Swedish MPA has asked an independent 'outside' expert to assess a drug product on its behalf, knowing that that scientist worked as a consultant on the product for the manufacturer and helped to prepare the manufacturer's application. When questioned as to the suitability of this arrangement, the response of the MPA official concerned with the assessment was that the agency was aware of the possible conflict of interest but knew the individual well and was content to allow them to advise the agency.[36] Although the practice raises a number of questions, it is not unusual for clinicians and other independent experts to work as consultants for pharmaceutical companies in addition to advising regulatory authorities. However, this is the only example we have uncovered where an agency deliberately utilised an outside expert who worked as a company consultant on the same product. Without greater transparency and openness, it is not possible to say whether this practice has occurred elsewhere. What the case may also highlight is the limited availability of independent experts who are knowledgeable in highly specialised therapeutic areas. As for the viability of expert advisors more generally, our findings suggest a recasting of advisory committee capacity to the European level, coupled with a diminution of influence at the national level.

## 'Independence' and conflicts of interest

Members of the CPMP are required to declare to the EMEA and the Commission any potential interests in the pharmaceutical industry within the preceding five years. The interests are defined according to the following four criteria:

- employment in the pharmaceutical industry;
- financial interests in the capital of a pharmaceutical company (e.g. shares);
- work currently or previously conducted by the member in return for payment, on behalf of the pharmaceutical industry;
- other interests which the member considers the EMEA ought to know about.

As explained in Chapter 4, there are thirty members of the CPMP – two members per Member State of the EU. In 1999, only one member of the CPMP declared current employment within the industry, one declared shares in a pharmaceutical company, four had received payment from the industry for various work, and four declared other interests, such as managing research institutes or co-ordinating clinical trials which were funded by pharmaceutical companies. It is immediately obvious that the extent of conflicts of interest declared by members of the CPMP is much less than is the case with members of the CSM (see Chapter 3).

This should not be surprising, because many members of the CPMP work for their national regulatory agencies rather than for expert advisory committees. In some EU countries, such as the UK, national regulators, as distinct from members of expert advisory committees, are not permitted to have any financial interests in the pharmaceutical industry. Both the British members of the CPMP are employed by the MCA, so they could not have any financial interests in the pharmaceutical industry. Thus, in this respect and, of course, in terms of decision-making power, the CPMP is more comparable to the MCA than the CSM. In short, the Europeanised body of experts, the CPMP, who are centrally involved in EU medicines regulation have significantly fewer conflicts of interest than national expert advisory committees, but more than many national regulatory agencies in the Union. Evidently, as at the national level, the 'independence' of expert scientists involved in medicines regulation is defined so as to permit personal and non-personal financial interests in the pharmaceutical industry.

## The global context of European regulatory science

The Europeanisation of medicines regulation is occurring, and at an accelerating pace. But harmonisation of regulatory standards and procedures in Europe is taking place within a wider context. The first International Conference on Harmonisation of Technical Requirements for Registration of Pharmaceuticals for Human Use (ICH) was convened in November 1991 in Brussels. The ICH is 'sponsored' by the regulatory authorities and pharmaceutical trade associations of the US, Japan and the EU. It has established itself as a major force in setting the agenda for drug testing requirements (Cone et al. 1992). While regulators attend meetings of the ICH, it is an industry-led organisation whose secretariat is provided by the International Federation of Pharmaceutical Industry Associations (IFPIA), and whose aim is to increase industrial efficiency by reducing the costs and burdens of drug testing. Nevertheless, the enthusiastic participation in and frequent support for ICH developments among regulators reveals the extent to which the neo-liberal political agenda has formulated and consolidated a corporatist, rather than adversarial, model of regulation transnationally.

This has had a marked impact on the science of drug testing. For example, in the field of repeat-dose toxicity testing in non-rodents, the FDA had required these tests to continue for 12 months, whereas the European regulatory authorities had accepted a repeat-dose toxicity test of merely 6 months duration, and continue to do so. The FDA believed that the European approach of 6-month toxicity tests in non-rodents was not adequate to detect some toxic effects. This was manifest during a controversy between the UK-based Centre for Medicines Research (CMR), funded by the ABPI, on the one hand, and the FDA, on the other. The FDA disputed the CMR's assertion that 12-month dog studies did not add any significant safety data.

Lack of consensus stemmed from the fact that the FDA defined significant findings as 'clinically significant toxicity ... serious enough to influence the design or progress of clinical trials' and necessitating 'regulatory action based on a reduced margin of safety' (Contrera *et al.* 1993: 65). By contrast, the CMR defined findings as 'significant' if they would 'influence the development of a compound' (Lumley *et al.* 1993: 54). Hence, the FDA defined 'significant' in terms of safety concerns and the need to intervene on the basis of those concerns, revealing the agency's awareness of its very public political environment of Congressional oversight, litigation and active consumer organisations. On the other hand, the CMR defined it in terms of the closed commercial world of whether the findings were so damaging to a prospective product that its industrial development was put in jeopardy. Evidently these different institutional perspectives influenced the definition of satisfactory standards for the science of drug testing.

The ICH was not able to persuade the FDA to replace its requirement for 12-month studies in dogs with 6-month studies for medicines intended for chronic use (Parkinson 1992). However, a compromise was reached at the ICH in July 1997 that 9-month tests were adequate, but European regulators remain free to accept 6-month studies (IFPIA 1998). Overall, therefore, the ICH recommended reduced testing requirements. Hence, this is an example of European regulators, the EMEA and the CPMP, altering the regulatory science of drug testing at the global level. It is important to appreciate that the global context of European harmonisation is not necessarily a constraining influence. On the contrary, the process of harmonisation is driven primarily from Europe.

This controversy illustrates how the institutional interests of industry and regulators expressed in harmonisation go right to the heart of the scientific uncertainty inherent in drug testing. That political factors were extremely important in framing the regulatory science in this case is supported by the comments of even those in industry who strongly support the move to reduce the duration of repeat-dose toxicity testing. For example, a knowledgeable official at EFPIA commented: 'I think that the most telling thing I could say is that it wasn't based on science – there probably isn't enough science to have anything based on it' (cited in Abraham and Reed 1998: 13).

While the ICH has been devoted to rationalising drug testing in the interests of industrial efficiency, it has shown little sign of developing harmonisation *aimed directly* at raising safety standards. Also underdeveloped within ICH work are discussions about comparative efficacy, which might lead to more efficient drug development but also probably higher standards of efficacy testing for the industry and, therefore, some cost increases. Thus, the efficiency drive of the ICH impacts upon the science of drug testing with a particular flavour and with considerable success by its own criteria. However, such success may be because of its exclusion of wider social groups in discussions of the development of drug testing. Issues and priorities that might provoke dissension in the wider social environment are transformed into areas of agreement by the bilateral industry–regulator context of the ICH. The disagreements between the FDA and the CMR are indications of just how much scope there could be for divergent opinions about scientific standards, if an even broader constituency of perspectives on drug safety were accommodated within these debates about regulatory medical science.

## The neglect of pharmacovigilance

The interplay between scientific expertise and political interests is as great in the area of pharmacovigilance as in pre-marketing assessment procedures. In Chapter 4, we explained why pharmacovigilance is becoming increasingly important within the European context. Given that the safety of new drugs can only be fully assessed after marketing, introduction of what are effectively European-wide approval systems means that the number of persons exposed to novel therapeutic treatments at the same time is likely to grow enormously. However, the social and political pressure for more adequate Europeanised pharmacovigilance cannot be merely translated into 'technical fixes'. *Politically*, the relationship between the national agencies and the European authorities (the EMEA and the CPMP) remains a thorny one, especially unilateral decisions by Member States to take local regulatory action against drug products which they consider to threaten public health. As noted in the previous chapter, a Member State should inform the EMEA and the CPMP if it is intending to suspend or withdraw a product licence, so that this can be co-ordinated at the European level. Such regulatory action is supposed to be permitted at the *national* level only on grounds of an urgent threat to public health. Despite this, in 1994 the German regulatory agency unilaterally suspended approval for one formulation of the anti-ulcer drug, omeprazole i/v bolus, because of its alleged carcinogenic risk (Anon 1994i). The CPMP criticised the German regulatory action, and eventually the suspension was lifted. This provoked condemnation from the German consumers' newsletter *aznei-telegramm*, which characterised the CPMP's stance as another indication that industrial interests take precedence over the obligation to protect consumers (Anon 1994k).

The global context is also important to understanding the 'science' of pharmacovigilance, which is increasingly a technocratic exercise in the control of information. Historically, the detection of ADRs has been facilitated by the WHO Programme for International Drug Monitoring, with the reporting of ADRs harmonised through initiatives by the Committee for the International Organisation of Medicines (CIOMS 1992; CIOMS 1990; WHO 1988). However, the Commission is obliged by EU law to establish separate procedures for monitoring the post-marketing safety of medicinal products in the Community (European Commission 1975b; 1993b: Title II, Chapter 3; 1995; EMEA 1999a). Nonetheless, despite this obligation, to date pharmacovigilance activity has taken second place to other concerns. As Professor Kjell Strandberg, Head of the Swedish MPA, has noted:

> Up to now, an overwhelming amount of time has of course been spent on the engineering of the new system for licensing purposes. Pharmacovigilance issues have come second to licensing issues. We now realise that in the EC context it will of course be more important to follow-up the drugs from a pharmacovigilance point of view on which we have taken joint licensing decisions.
>
> (Anon 1995g: 1006)

The failure to confront the issue of post-marketing surveillance and to devote more resources to it has meant that the Commission has come under increasing pressure to improve pharmacovigilance standards from both the European Parliament and European consumer organisations. To this end, one or more national reference centres have been established in each Member State and improvements are being made to inter-agency communications through greater use of information technology systems. According to the Commission, the latter will enable 'direct links between pharmacovigilance and decision-making' to be introduced, although exactly how these links will operate in practice and the effect they are likely to have is hard to discern. The aim is to replace paper reporting by electronic transfer of information between EU bodies, national authorities and companies, irrespective of the authorisation procedure used. To this end, the EMEA and the EFPIA have agreed to streamline reporting, with formation of a Joint Pilot Group to trial electronic transmission of individual patient case reports (EMEA 1999d). The development of electronic transmission of ADR information also highlights the push for harmonisation of medical terminology through programmes such as the Medical Dictionary for Regulatory Activities (MEDDRA), now adopted for use across the EU, and globally by the ICH (D'Arcy and Harron 1996: 495–8).

Implementation of improved pharmacovigilance standards, however, is not solely a 'technical matter'. It is affected by cultural aspects involving differences in the practice of medicine in Member States as well as by (uncertain) science. Strandberg, for example, foresees problems arising from the huge cultural differences existing in Europe, primarily because there has been no forum in which to deal with such problems on a joint basis, as there has been for licensing issues (Anon 1995g). The interface between EU and national political responsibilities for public health is especially relevant here. Nevertheless, like pre-marketing systems, pharmacovigilance systems in Europe are being developed jointly by industry and regulators, with little or no participation by other interests. This has led to the creation of what one industry spokesperson describes as: 'a sort of club of specialists in pharmacovigilance ... bringing together representatives of the universities as well as industry and the health authorities' (Juillett 1994: 39).

According to public pronouncements, neither the European Commission nor the Council of Ministers consider the present systems adequate. Fernand Sauer, Head of the EMEA, has stated that deficiencies include the non-availability of information, difficulties in the medical and cultural perception of certain classes of medicine, differences in scientific assessment between authorities, and unilateral decisions sometimes made by Member States (Anon 1993j). Specific plans to combat these problems include making each Member State establish a system for collecting and evaluating ADR reports, and optimising the exchange of information. To this end, in 1993 the Commission funded a group under Sir Michael Rawlins, a former chairman of the British CSM and now director of the UK National Institute for Clinical Excellence (NICE), to set up the European Pharmacovigilance Research Group (EPVRG). The group's brief was to examine the strengths and weaknesses of existing post-marketing surveillance systems in Europe and develop ways of improving ADR reporting.

In practical terms, the EU has opted to develop its own ADR reporting network, using the MCA's MEDDRA. Reporting systems will be highly automated, with database-to-database communication involving minimal human intervention. Reports will be channelled through the national competent authorities' reporting systems to prevent or reduce double counting, while industry will be encouraged to centralise internal ADR reporting procedures. However, the adoption of specifically EU systems has also brought the Commission into conflict with the WHO over ADR reporting systems, despite the fact that the two bodies have established a collaborative programme, and that collaboration is laid down in EU law (European Commission 1993a). In fact, WHO scientists have generally felt marginalised in an area where the organisation has many years' experience and similar, if geographically and politically broader, interests.[37]

The Commission adopted the view that the WHO reporting system (WHOART) was out of date and under intense competition from systems developed by the US (COSTART) and the UK (ADROIT), while the Japanese seldom used WHOART. The WHO argued that their reporting system could have been built upon and improved in order to satisfy all parties, including the EU. One argument advanced is that the EU has effectively created a separate and competing reporting system for political-bureaucratic, rather than scientific, reasons. Whatever the validity of this argument, the WHO reporting system has been generally ignored. However, the Commission rejects the suggestion that it is duplicating services already provided by WHO, stressing the need to distinguish between legal reporting requirements specified in EU law and the medical terminology system used, of which the WHO system is one among several.[38] Recently, in an effort to improve and clarify relations, the EMEA has released a set of principles on providing pharmacovigilance information to the WHO (EMEA 1998a).

From the perspective of national standards, pharmacovigilance systems vary considerably between Member States. To date, responsibility has been largely left to national authorities, with the CPMP sometimes intervening. In the future, regulators believe the integrity of national systems will have to be maintained within an over-arching EU network co-ordinated by the CPMP. As discussed in the following chapter, even if local pre-market assessment capability disappears, all States will be obliged to maintain the capacity to conduct pharmacovigilance for political reasons. Some regulators argue that because the pharmacovigilance system is much more reliant on national experts than pre-market testing, more detailed guidelines are called for. Various guidelines and procedures have indeed been introduced, including a rapid alert system and a drug information monitoring scheme. However, many of the rapid alerts issued since 1989 either failed to meet the criteria for an alert or have generated little action. According to the then chairman of the EU Working Group on Pharmacovigilance, they had disappeared into a 'dark pit', while overall output from the Working Party itself was characterised as 'disappointing' (Wood 1996; EMEA 1997b, 1999a).

The variation in Member States' standards regarding pharmacovigilance was illustrated in the case of Ketorolac.[39] In April 1994, when there was wide disagreement among Member States on the scientific interpretation of the data and the course of action demanded by it, the CPMP gave an opinion on the anti-inflammatory drug. On this occasion, the CPMP satisfied all participants in the dispute by allowing different interpretations to be placed on the evidence, in accordance with members' wishes. Following the submission of additional safety data by the manufacturer, the CPMP declared that the product had a narrow therapeutic margin (meaning that its risk/benefit ratio was small). When used in accordance with restrictions the Committee had issued the previous year, the benefit/risk ratio was deemed acceptable in Belgium, Denmark, Italy, Luxembourg, Spain and the UK. But a marketing authorisation could not be granted in Ireland until results of a study on comparative safety and efficacy were submitted and evaluated. Even when used in accordance with the same restrictions noted above, the product was *not* considered adequate by France, Germany, Greece, the Netherlands and Portugal. The CPMP action provides a definitive demonstration of the extent of disagreement between Member States at the post-marketing stage prior to the introduction of 'binding' CPMP arbitration (Anon 1994e).

But has the position changed as regards pharmacovigilance issues brought before the CPMP since the establishment of the 'strong' regulatory state in 1995? The UK government's unilateral decision in 1996 to issue warnings of a link between so-called 'third generation' oral contraceptives and increased thrombosis-like events without first seeking CPMP agreement suggests there remains considerable room for independent action. In this case, the UK authority (in the form of the CSM) unilaterally issued statements to the media concerning possible long-term health risks to certain groups of women taking the drug, and advised British doctors not to prescribe certain brands to some women. Subsequently, the CPMP downplayed the significance of the reported risks and issued advice counter to that of the UK agency.

## Conclusion

Europeanisation of medicines regulation is occurring, and at an accelerating pace. Yet a European 'superstate' of medicines regulation, akin to the American FDA, remains a 'virtual reality' without the resources to develop a substantial independent base of regulatory scientists. While Europeanisation of medicines regulation is real and perhaps more rapid than in any other sector, it remains fundamentally dependent on the expertise and resources derived from the national agencies. In these respects the combined regulatory power of the Commission, the EMEA and the CPMP is much less autonomous than that of the FDA, even though the EU *en bloc* now represents the largest market for pharmaceuticals in the world.

Nevertheless, harmonisation is meeting with greater success under the new regime than previously, not because the drug products manufactured by the industry suddenly command the approval of regulatory scientists across Europe, but rather because of political, bureaucratic and institutional changes which have induced regulators to compromise and reach consensus. Having said this, these changes have partly involved a reformulation of scientific expertise from the national to the European level – changes that have been further facilitated by the more global efforts to harmonise scientific standards of drug testing and pharmacovigilance by the ICH since 1991.

One of the most significant political forces behind European harmonisation is the convergence of institutional interests between national agencies and the industry in rapid drug approvals. In particular, the mutual recognition system that has been established involves national regulatory authorities within the EU competing with each other for regulatory work provided by fees from the pharmaceutical industry. This competition puts pressure on the national authorities to 'sell themselves' as the fastest in reviewing and approving drugs. Ironically, this Europeanised system of medicines regulation has created conflicts of interest between the national agencies within the EU.

When viewed mechanistically and in isolation, both the centralised and decentralised procedures involve greater scientific peer review of regulatory assessments, among Member States and/or at the EU level. At least superficially, this ought to improve regulatory decision-making. However, these procedures should not be divorced from the broader and much more complex political context of Europeanised medicines regulation. This is because, first, the pressure of rapid regulatory review may undermine that very peer review, as Concerned Member States do not have the time to check thoroughly the evaluation of the Reference Member State. And second, that very peer review, combined with compressed timeframes, is leading to a diminished role for national expert science advisory committees, who have themselves provided an important 'independent' form of peer review. Our findings imply that, from 1998, some expert science advisory committees are likely to become less independent from the national agencies whom they advise, as expert advisers are integrated into specific problem areas of risk-benefit assessment early in the regulatory review process. Others are likely to be absorbed into EU expert advisory functions to an even greater extent than at present.

Our research confirms the view that decision-making about medicines regulation is not *solely* a matter of technical science. Rather, medicines regulation *also* involves social and political judgements. To some readers, this will come as no surprise. However, the problem for the European drug regulatory systems is that their *official representation* is of purely scientific processes. It is on this basis that the delegation of medicines regulation to technical scientists is justified by European governments. The drive to improve and harmonise pharmacovigilance is also becoming increasing specialist and technocratic. Solutions are thought to reside almost entirely in more sophisticated and precise terminology and better management of data systems, and much less in the involvement of the wider medical community and health professionals/advocates. However, our research has revealed the contradictions of these scientistic representations of European harmonisation. The influence of institutional and political interests on the Europeanisation of medicines regulation is very much in evidence – some of which may penetrate deeply into regulatory science. This raises fundamental questions about whether European medicines control should continue along its technocratic route of relying entirely on scientists to reach regulatory decisions, or whether the process should be made more democratic by allowing a broader range of social interests to have some input into European medicines regulation – an issue to which we return at greater length in Chapter 7.

# Chapter 6

# Competition, harmonisation and public health

An issue of major importance for all concerned is whether the new Europeanised system of medicines regulation will improve public health by promoting the development of safer drugs on to the market or compromise it by permitting patients to be exposed to hazardous drug products, which might have been rejected or withdrawn under the former national systems of regulation. Assessments of drug safety are often difficult for regulatory agencies, who have to weigh up a complex array of risks and benefits for patients in a context of incomplete information and scientific uncertainty. Moreover, as we have argued in previous chapters, medicines regulation is not a purely scientific process. Rather, scientific uncertainties are compounded – and sometimes even produced – by commercial, professional and institutional interests. Thus, the challenge for a supranational European regulatory system to harmonise the protection of public health adequately is formidable.

## Halcion, Viagra and other disharmonies

Nowhere was the challenge to harmonisation more evident than in the pan-European controversy over the safety of the sleeping pill, Halcion (triazolam). On 2 October 1991, the UK regulatory authorities suspended Halcion from the British market on the grounds that it was a threat to public health because its risks of serious adverse psychiatric effects outweighed its benefits (Gabe and Bury 1996). Since then, it has remained banned in the UK (Abraham and Sheppard 1998). However, about a week after the suspension of Halcion in the UK, the chairman of the EU's CPMP, then Professor Poggiolini, wrote to all the other Member State regulatory authorities asking them not to take any action against Halcion until the CPMP had discussed the situation (Anon 1991i). Later in October 1991, the CPMP expressed concern that the British regulatory authorities had acted unilaterally without discussing their intention to withdraw Halcion with other EU Member States. Rather than withdraw the product from EU markets, the CPMP set up a working party to examine the safety of Halcion further (Anon 1991; 1991l). From the perspective of the MCA, this decision extended the period during which patients were exposed to a dangerous drug, while Bermuda, Finland, Jamaica and Norway followed the British example by suspending the product on their markets (Anon 1991c).

It was not only the British regulators who presented problems for European harmonisation in the Halcion case. In December 1991, the CPMP's working group on Halcion, including two eminent German regulators, recommended that the drug should be withdrawn throughout the EU, but the full Committee did not accept this recommendation (Anon 1992c). The drug was available in the EU in two tablet forms reflecting an upper and lower daily dosage for patients. Rejecting the conclusions of its working party, the CPMP decided not to recommend the withdrawal of the product in either of its dosage forms (Anon 1991n). However, within a month, the French Pharmacovigilance Commission recommended that the Health Ministry of France should suspend the product because of its adverse effects on patients. Contrary to the CPMP's recommendation, the French Health Ministry responded by removing the higher dose tablet from the market in France (Anon 1992b).

A similar story may be told about the intravenous version of the anti-ulcer drug, Losec (omeprazole). It was associated with almost a hundred reports of visual disorders in patients in the EU, forty-seven of the reports being in Germany (Anon 1994h). Consequently, in August 1994 the German regulatory authorities suspended the marketing approval for intravenous Losec on safety grounds, even though, just a few weeks earlier, the CPMP had rejected any suggestion that the drug should be removed from the market, because the Committee was not convinced that the data available established a causal link between Losec and severe visual disorders (Anon 1994i; 1994j). During the same summer, the Spanish Health Ministry revoked the licence of the non-steroidal anti-inflammatory drug Ombolan (droxicam) because of its association with reports of liver damage, in contradiction with the CPMP's opinion that withdrawal of the product on safety grounds was unnecessary (Anon 1994g).

As the CPMP's marketing authorisation opinions became binding on EU Member States in 1995, disharmony over safety judgements continued. The British regulatory authorities took unilateral action to limit the use of seven brands of 'third generation' oral contraceptives on safety grounds. After reviewing several epidemiological studies of 'third generation' oral contraceptives containing the progestogens gestodene or desogestrel, the CSM concluded that those contraceptives were associated with an increase in the incidence of thrombo-embolism (venous thrombosis) compared with 'second generation' pills (Anon 1995h). Consequently, they advised doctors to switch all women on the 'third generation' products to other brands (Anon 1997n). Norway took the same action as the British, while the German regulatory agency prohibited prescription of the offending brands to first-time users of the pill who were under 30 years of age. However, other regulatory agencies in the EU disagreed, and in a position statement issued by the EMEA, the CPMP indicated that they thought the epidemiological studies were flawed in design and did not warrant the cessation of marketing the products across Europe (EMEA 1995a). As with Halcion, the British regulators were condemned by some of their European counterparts for taking precipitate action, while other observers questioned whether the EU was being too complacent about the safety of patients.

The question of whether the EU's regulatory system is complacent about public safety is particularly significant within the centralised procedure, which may result in decisions which expose millions of patients across Europe to a new drug in a very short period. For example, the innovative oral impotence pill Viagra (sildenafil), for which Pfizer sought marketing approval via the centralised procedure, was estimated to have a market of over 5 million patients suffering from erectile dysfunction in Spain and Italy alone (Anon 1998j). When the drug was approved in the US in March 1998, it was being prescribed at a rate of 20,000 per day (Anon 1998e). Between April and June 1998, a total of 2.9 million prescriptions were written for the drug (Anon 1998m). Two months later, the CPMP recommended that Viagra should be approved for marketing across the EU – a market similar in size to the US – despite emerging safety concerns across the Atlantic (Anon 1998i).

Viagra seems to offer significant benefits for some, perhaps many, patients. In that sense, it is a genuine therapeutic innovation. On the other hand, during the clinical trials with Viagra, about 150 (3 per cent) of the 4,500 men tested experienced visual disturbances, consisting of light sensitivity and a blue colouring of vision. Pfizer are confident that the 'blue vision effect' is transient and has no lasting effect on the eye or the retina (Anon 1998h). However, in May 1998 some American ophthalmologists warned that the long-term implications of the adverse visual effects were unknown, and expressed concern that Viagra could cause permanent vision loss in patients already suffering from retinal dysfunction. It was also noted by a professor of ophthalmology at Stanford University that about 10 per cent of people taking the higher recommended dose had reported the 'blue vision effect' (Anon 1998h).

Moreover, in July 1998 the FDA reported that Viagra had been associated with 77 deaths since marketing in the US, but for 24 of these the information was unverifiable. Of the remainder, the cause of death is known for 26 – two had strokes and 24 had cardiac events, such as 'heart attack'. Fourteen died, or developed symptoms that led to death, within two hours of sexual activity (Anon 1998p). In response, the Chairman of Pharmacology at Georgetown University in Washington DC warned that Viagra may increase cardiotoxicity by interacting with drugs which lower blood pressure, and the American public health advocacy group, Public Citizen, argued that it should be contraindicated for patients with a history of strokes or cardiac failure because such patients were excluded from clinical trials (Anon 1998l).

Nevertheless, in September 1998 the European Commission accepted the CPMP's advice on Viagra and approved the drug for marketing authorisation throughout the EU. While the nature and extent of Viagra's direct effects on patients' health remain to be seen, the Commission's decision posed drug regulatory problems with indirect effects on public health in some Member States (Anon 1998u). In the UK, an immediate problem was the implica-tion for other public health provision if the National Health Service (NHS) had to pay for millions of Viagra prescriptions. To offset this difficulty, the British Health Secretary sought to manage demand for Viagra by restricting its prescription and declaring that doctors' prescriptions would only be reimbursed by the NHS for patients who 'clinically needed' the drug (Anon 1998n).

In September 1998, the UK Department of Health sent a circular to NHS doctors advising them not to prescribe Viagra 'save in exceptional circumstances' (Anon 1999c). However, Pfizer challenged the legality of the circular in the UK High Court in May 1999. The judge found in the company's favour, concluding that the Health Secretary could not lawfully deter doctors from complying with their statutory obligation to prescribe a drug for which there is a clinical need when the drug is not included on the NHS 'black list', Schedule 10 (products that are not available on the NHS because they are expensive and of questionable therapeutic value). The implications of this ruling went well beyond Viagra. The UK National Institute for Clinical Excellence (NICE) was set up to advise doctors about therapeutically efficient prescribing, especially on when and whether to prescribe various drugs, without placing them on Schedule 10 (Anon 1999a). According to its chairman, the UK Department of Health expected advice from NICE to be followed 'to the letter'. Yet the Viagra court ruling implies that such advice could be unlawful. Thus, the European centralised licensing of Viagra seems to have set in train a series of events which have undermined the British government's autonomy in managing medicines within its national healthcare system.

The examples above show that concerns about the safety of medicines vary among experts in different national contexts, and that questions about whether the EU's new system of medicines regulation will increase or decrease drug safety have very real consequences for patients' exposure to dangerous drugs and/or their access to important therapeutic innovations. Disagreements about drug safety, such as those over Halcion or 'third generation' oral contraceptives, usually enter the public arena after a drug is marketed, but they often relate to how safety was evaluated prior to marketing approval. In other words, there is much more to the harmonisation of drug safety withdrawals than solely the harmonisation of pharmacovigilance. Moreover, as the approval process is the main mechanism employed to check medicines for safety and to protect public health, we concentrate on that in this chapter.

While it is patients who are affected by how the safety of medicines is regulated, the main actors involved in the regulatory process are scientists and regulatory affairs managers in industry and governmental regulatory agencies. Critics and consumer organisations claim that too often the national drug regulatory systems that have been established around the world do not safeguard public health sufficiently (Chetley 1995; Medawar 1992a; Mintzes and Hodgkin 1996; Moore 1995; Pearce 1996). Furthermore, in the context of Canadian drug regulation, Lexchin has raised two further related concerns: that regulators excessively accommodate the interests of the pharmaceutical industry at the expense of patients' interests in safety, because their relationship with drug companies is 'too close for comfort' (1990: 1257); and that governmental efforts to hasten drug approval 'could jeopardize safety considerations' (1994: 257). These are important matters which are also relevant to the new EU-wide regulatory procedures for medicines. On the other hand, an optimistic view put forward by Davis (1997: 145) is that 'international harmonisation of standards and regulatory processes, if managed correctly, could both strengthen safety regimes, and speed approvals of new drugs'. To examine these important issues in more depth, we asked many of the main actors from government and industry in the EU for their perspectives on the impact of European harmonisation on safety standards, regulator–industry interactions and approval times in relation to safety.

## Safety standards

The vast majority of industrial scientists and regulatory affairs managers in industry believed that European harmonisation would either raise safety standards or at least maintain them as high as previous national standards (Table 6.1). Some respondents in industry thought this because they believed harmonisation is 'rationalising' scientific standards for safety evaluation:

> Well, if anything, it's been a 'levelling up'; there's never been a 'levelling down'. I think the only thing that you could expect is possibly a more rational approach to scientific standards, and I think we're getting that to an extent. We're sorting out the real scientific issues from the national, cultural differences.[1]

As one regulatory affairs manager acknowledged, this 'rationalisation' involves discarding some toxicity testing but, he argued, without lowering safety standards because those tests are superfluous:

> Harmonisation will lead to less ridiculous requirements hopefully. Normally my experience is that they [regulators and other standard-setters] do not agree on a lower standard. The

Table 6.1   Industry and regulator views on potential levelling down of
safety standards ('There is, or is likely to be, a levelling
down of safety standards')

|  | n | No (%) | Yes (%) | Unsure (%) |
|---|---|---|---|---|
| Industry | 27 | 24 (89) | 2  (7) | 1  (4) |
| UK regulators | 2 | 1  (50) | 1 (50) | 0  (0) |
| German regulators | 4 | 2 (50) | 2 (50) | 0  (0) |
| Swedish regulators | 7 | 1  (14) | 4 (57) | 2 (29) |
| EU regulators | 2 | 2 (100) | 0  (0) | 0  (0) |
| Totals | 42 | 30  (71) | 9 (22) | 3  (7) |

requirement is always higher than before. What is also a fact
is that the unnecessary burden of safety testing is reduced. So
we don't have to do what we did in the past just because it
was a requirement, rather than because it is scientifically justified. This is not a risk to public health.[2]

Even one of the two respondents from industry who agreed that
safety standards were being lowered by harmonisation also
remarked that the peer review among Member States within the
mutual recognition procedure could raise safety standards:

There can be a raising of standards in other Member States. If
you submit an application to the UK, and they are just
approving it nationally, nothing to do with Europe, then I do
believe that you have an easier time, and there is a different
assessment done too if you are going into a mutual recognition procedure because the MCA is conscious of the fact that
it is going to have to defend its decisions and its judgement,
and consequently it is more critical of its own judgement, and
therefore makes the job a bit harder.[3]

By contrast, no such consensus existed among the regulators we
interviewed. In fact, a slight majority of them believed that EU
harmonisation was likely to lead to a 'levelling downwards' of
safety standards (Table 6.1). Two German regulators were
unequivocal about this:

*Interviewer:*    Are you saying that there are instances where either
                  this authority [BfArM] or other national authorities
                  in the EU have had to or have accepted a product
                  which, under their own national procedures, they
                  would not normally have done?
*BfArM2:*         Of course.
*Interviewer:*    Which then, potentially anyway, does lead to a
                  lowering of safety standards, by definition?
*BfArM2:*         Of course.[4]

The other was sceptical about the whole project of harmonisation
regarding drug safety. He viewed it as being driven by commercial
and trade interests rather than concerns about safety regulation:

> Benefiting safety is not the goal of European harmonisation.
> Harmonisation on the drug level is part of the commercial
> part of the EU – the single market – DGIII [the EU Directive
> for trade and industry] is dealing with the problem. It's about
> access to the market, not to benefit safety.[5]

On the reasonable assumption that there is a danger that trade
and industry interests might subordinate health and safety needs
(Anon 1997f), then there is evidence to support this regulator's
view from within the European Commission and Parliament. In
January 1997, a European parliamentary committee argued that
the Commission's public protection powers and responsibilities
should be brought under DGXXIV (the consumer affairs direc-
torate) because it is not 'directly liable to pressure from industrial
interests' (Anon 1997a). Speaking before this committee, Jacques
Santer, then President of the Commission, implied that EMEA
might be switched to DGXXIV. However, this has not occurred.
   Swedish regulators echoed concerns about the impact of
Europeanisation on safety standards:

*Interviewer:*    Are you optimistic that safety standards will be main-
                  tained under European harmonisation?
*MPA2:*           I think we were better off before.
*Interviewer:*    Why?
*MPA2:*           Because we had the knowledge, we had the experi-
                  ence, we had the rulings and I don't think that we
                  have any bad examples of our handling of this, and I

think Europe has learned a lot from us, and I don't think we have much to gain from them.[6]

The British regulator who believed that safety standards would be harmonised downwards acknowledged that safety standards might be raised in some Member States:

> I think that the UK has always had a very high standard for new chemical entities and bio-tech products [NASs]. So I think for us it's inevitably going to mean a 'levelling down' from our perspective. Now for others [other Member States] it may well be a 'levelling up'.[7]

Furthermore, this MCA scientist expressed concern that the European procedures would require them to approve 'rather mediocre products where the clinical benefit is not clear'.[8] One of the expert scientific advisers to the MPA also approached these procedures with trepidation:

> Sweden is much tougher for the companies than some other European countries. We are afraid that the Swedish market could be flooded with a number of drugs that we do not really want to have because we do not know enough about their pharmacokinetics, adverse reactions in patients, interactions with other drugs and so on.[9]

While both of the regulators working at the EU level rejected the suggestion that safety standards might be lowered by European harmonisation, only one of the seven Swedish regulators interviewed was confident that it would raise safety standards because of the additional scientific expertise brought to bear on the issue across Europe:

> I think there's a levelling up. The standards have been raised all over. That's why it is my view that [harmonisation] will not have a major impact on public health in Sweden ... if there is lower competence by some Member States within a specific area, that means that they will not be involved so much in the assessment, evaluation, discussions and so on, in the decision-making on that particular product because that will be led by those that have the expertise.[10]

## Approval times, inter-agency competition and safety evaluation

As we explained in Chapter 4, in order to further the goal of a single pharmaceutical market in Europe and to accommodate the industry's desire for more rapid approval times, since 1 January 1995 strict timescales have been prescribed by the European Commission for the mutual recognition procedure. Regulatory agencies in the EU are funded to a greater or lesser extent by fees for their regulatory work paid by the industry. In particular, the largest amount of regulatory work (and hence fees) is generated by Reference Member State status within the mutual recognition procedure – rapporteur status in the centralised procedure comes a poor second. Such status is also important to the regulatory agencies because it represents much more interesting and challenging scientific work than the 'checking' role that comes with Concerned Member State status. By maximising its Reference Member State or rapporteur work, a national regulatory agency increases the likelihood of keeping and attracting good-quality scientists. Hence, because the agencies of Member States now compete for 'regulatory business', they are under considerable pressure to conform to these snappy timetables, especially as companies look for fast approval rates as one of their key criteria when choosing a Reference Member State.

Also of particular significance for safety evaluation is the fact that, under the mutual recognition procedure, a marketing authorisation in one Member State ought to be recognised by other Member States unless there are 'grounds for supposing that the authorisation may present a risk to public health' (European Commission 1996a: 7). If a Member State cannot accept an authorisation of another Member State, it must immediately inform the company, the Reference Member State, the Concerned Member States and the CPMP, stating the reasons for its decision and indicating how the gaps in the application might be filled. A compulsory conciliation stage then follows to facilitate the Member State's recognition of the Reference Member State's authorisation (Deboyser 1996b: 117). Thus, regulators are under pressure to adopt quickly a position on the Reference Member State authorisation and to assemble robust evidence to support that position, if they propose to reject the authorisation on grounds of risk to public health. As one scientist at the MPA acknowledged:

*Interviewer:* You seem to be implying that the Europeanisation process is putting pressure on the MPA, and perhaps other EU regulatory agencies, to approve drugs?

*MPA6:* Yes.

*Interviewer:* But you're not saying there is any pressure in the other direction – pressure to be more strict in approving drugs. Is that a fair summary?

*MPA6:* That's a fair summary of my concerns, yes.[11]

Pressure from industry on regulators to harmonise their assessments of drug safety has continued unabated. In May 1998, the EFPIA claimed that industry's confidence in the mutual recognition procedure remained low because of the inconsistencies in regulators' interpretation of 'significant public health issues' in different Member States (Anon 1998g). Within two months, the MRFG had implemented new procedures intended to help resolve public health concerns raised by Member States so that marketing approval could be harmonised more effectively (Anon 1998k). This would seem to give support to the perception that Europeanisation gives rise to pressure to approve drugs rather than reject them.

Representatives of the industry welcome inter-agency competition and believe that it leads to both higher quality regulatory assessments of drug applications and faster approvals. For example, a senior EFPIA official commented:

> I think the competition is to be welcomed because [regulators] have to prove that [they're] better, not just faster. And companies are going to choose that Member State that not only gets them a fast opinion but that ensures that that is acceptable throughout Europe.[12]

Similarly, the vast majority of our respondents from industry did not think that this inter-agency competition posed a threat to public health by undercutting the quality of safety evaluation (Table 6.2). In some cases the MCA has claimed that it can complete the assessment of an application, including safety evaluation, in much less than 210 days – one well-publicised example being a 53-day assessment. However, when it was put to industry sources that this competition might undermine safety, they generally challenged the proposition that fast approvals implied lower quality regulation as follows:

I don't think that you can generally say, how can they [regulators] assess this product in 53 days, because it could be that they have just recently gone through a very similar compound and they knew exactly what they should look at ... Time limit, fair or not, depends upon the competence within the authorities and the resources they have.[13]

As Table 6.2 shows, overall the regulators were evenly split on this question. Five were confident that inter-agency competition for industry fees does not threaten public health, five felt that it does, and five conceded that it might. Neither of the British regulators or the EU regulators thought that such competition posed a threat to public health. In fact, most of them believed that competition between regulatory authorities had created beneficial peer review among Member States. They rejected the proposition that such competitive pressure encourages regulators to 'cut corners' in safety evaluation:

A number of people said, okay, you [the MCA] are fast, but how do we know that your quality is okay? Our answer ... is that we [the MCA] could not afford to be as stupid as that. That's the first basic commercial thing. The second thing is that we have obviously got a professional reputation to uphold ... And in the centralised process there is peer review because if we're the reference member state and the company is going to roll our authorisation on to other countries [Member States], we've got to provide an assessment report that stands up to their [other Member States'] scrutiny.[14]

*Table 6.2*    Industry and regulator views on competition between Member States as a threat to public health ('Competition between Member States is a threat to public health')

|                    | n  | No (%)    | Yes (%) | Possibly (%) |
|--------------------|----|-----------|---------|--------------|
| Industry           | 27 | 22 (81)   | 2 (7)   | 3 (12)       |
| UK regulators      | 2  | 1 (50)    | 0 (0)   | 1 (50)       |
| German regulators  | 4  | 2 (50)    | 1 (25)  | 1 (25)       |
| Swedish regulators | 7  | 0 (0)     | 4 (57)  | 3 (43)       |
| EU regulators      | 2  | 2 (100)   | 0 (0)   | 0 (0)        |
| Totals             | 42 | 27 (64)   | 7 (17)  | 8 (19)       |

Some German regulators echoed these views:

> You can only survive the [European] system if what you are
> doing is scientifically sound. If you are doing anybody [i.e. a
> company] a favour, this might work on a purely national
> basis, but the moment you go into the European arena, you
> will have to explain this to others and this will be very diffi-
> cult ... now most [BfArM] experts have learned to defend
> their views in open discussions with other experts brought in
> by industry, and this has improved the whole level of our
> assessment. This is not a move in the direction of making it
> easier for industry, in some respects it's even the opposite, but
> in some respects it's on a better, higher level now.[15]

However, one medical assessor at the MCA conceded that inter-
agency competition creates a tension for regulators:

> I mean we are in a difficult position. Of course, we want
> people to apply with national applications to us [i.e. Reference
> Member State status] because that's how we get our, that's
> how we survive – fee-based. But we won't do it at the expense
> of prostituting ourselves.[16]

Worries about that tension were articulated much more force-
fully and pervasively by Swedish regulators. It is particularly
notable that *none* of our respondents at the MPA felt confident
that inter-agency competition would not threaten public health.
Specifically, some Swedish regulators showed concern that competition between agencies and pressure to reduce approval times at
the behest of industry might undermine the quality of safety and
efficacy evaluations. As one MPA scientist explained:

> I'm a bit concerned when I see agencies like the MCA market
> themselves as being the quickest, 65 days or 54 days. I think
> it's a pity if we as agencies start running in a race which the
> industry might like, but we tend to forget why we have agen-
> cies. Agencies are there to make sure that safe and effective
> drugs are on the market – as consumer protection. The health-
> care systems are less interested in 56 or 86 days, they're more
> interested in the quality of the assessment. And I think it's a
> bit unfortunate that we, together with all the other agencies,

have not been able to say: OK, time is now decided at 210 days. That's what we have to work with, we accept that, but let's not race faster than that. Let's make the best out of those days. Instead of competing, let's make the best evaluations instead of the quickest ones.[17]

Moreover, when asked if competition between agencies could mean that the EU was moving to a regulatory system based on the lowest common denominator – that is, a 'levelling down' in standards rather than a 'levelling up' – this MPA scientist commented:

Yes, that's the fear. I'm sure the industry wants to avoid the highest one, if by highest you mean the most complicated hurdles to have a drug approved. What we want to avoid is that we end up with a situation where it's too easy and there's nothing negative about it. It's that fear that we're not picking out the rotten eggs, the problems.[18]

Other Swedish regulators were also concerned that inter-agency competition for ever faster approval could result in important safety matters being overlooked:

The time limits as they are set now [210 days] are very tight and to reduce them further would really endanger the whole system of putting safe drugs on the market.[19]

There's a risk involved with this that some matters have been handled rapidly. I think it would be better that we didn't have that pressure upon us. I think it would be better for the companies too because it's not good for them to have products on the market which must be withdrawn because we have missed something here.[20]

The German regulator, who believed that these competitive pressures threatened public health, was particularly concerned that the drive for fast approvals would lead to excessive trust being invested in the documentation submitted by manufacturers:

If you try to assess complicated products in a very short time, in most cases you must believe what is written down by companies. If you have a company working correctly, it's not a problem, but if you have companies which are not, there will be a problem. To find these companies out you must have time. I think there will be a risk for safety in the future.[21]

In November 1997, some of these concerns voiced by regulators about rapid drug approvals in the EU seemed to be given support by Professor Silvio Garattini, a member of the CPMP. He claimed that most products submitted to the EU's centralised procedure were 'me-too' drugs, and that too many products were approved 'prematurely', pending the completion of clinical trials (Anon 1997l). According to Garattini, only 16 per cent of products submitted to the centralised procedure were 'really new'. He suggested that more comparative clinical trials showing benefits over existing products should be required by the CPMP and the EMEA. The implication of his proposal is that safety evaluation should be harmonised upwards by taking more account of comparative safety and efficacy in EU medicines regulation.

In the German context, the extent to which the MCA and the MPA are dependent on fees from industry was sometimes heavily criticised for distorting regulatory assessments against the public interest. For example, a senior scientist at BfArM commented:

We are fee-based, but this covers less than half our income so the interests of the public are also represented in our fee system. We are not so easily put under pressure from industry. He who pays the piper calls the tune – it is said. This is also true in our business, and having a certain independence is reflected in the work we do. If you [a regulatory agency] go decentralised [i.e. take on RMS status] you get the full national fee but, because of the role of EMEA in the centralised procedure, you get less than that if you go centralised. The MCA and MPA advise everybody to use the decentralised system because otherwise they would lose enormous amounts of money. So that puts those agencies under pressure that we don't have.[22]

Even a regulatory affairs manager of a German-based company voiced concerns about the pressure on regulatory agencies to generate fees from industry:

There is a down side. This is that as soon as the regulators need a certain income, the money has to really flow in, and if their decision to fight for a product, to get the application, is based on the calculation of money and not anything else, it would be a disaster, and that has started already with the MCA. And other authorities are fighting for the decentralised mutual recognition procedure in cases where the centralised procedure would be more feasible, just because of the money.[23]

Certainly, the financial viability of some national regulatory agencies in the EU seems to balance finely on fees from companies for regulatory work. For example, the MCA sought to receive £27 million of its income from industry fees in 1999 to meet its operating costs, involving a fee of about £55,000 to review a product under the mutual recognition procedure (Anon 1998w). While the distortion of advice to companies about which Euro-procedure to follow does not necessarily undermine safety evaluation, another senior scientist at BfArM explicitly connected agencies' financial independence to the maintenance of drug safety:

> To hold the safety and quality aspects you need such independent institutes like the German one. The German regulators have no risk to their jobs so they can decide solely by scientific, and not other reasons. I think there is a big risk that agencies like the MCA and MPA are losing their independence.[24]

## Industry–regulator closeness and consultation

The credibility of European regulators in the eyes of those who see them as being 'too close' to industry was not helped by allegations in 1993 that Professor Poggiolini, then chairman of the CPMP, had received numerous 'costly gifts' from over a dozen pharmaceutical companies during his twenty years at the Italian Health Ministry (Anon 1993n). It was reported that, after investigators raided his house and questioned him about more than a hundred paintings and works of art found there, Poggiolini stated that, during the 1980s, 'the custom of exchanging costly gifts was widespread and tolerated, if not condoned, by everyone' (Anon 1993n: 3). In his testimony, he proceeded to name the pharmaceutical companies involved. Poggiolini alleged that the value of the gifts ranged from $6,200 from one company to $310,000 from another.

While conflicts of interest within the CPMP have become less pronounced than the Poggiolini case suggests (see Chapter 5), consultation and, arguably, participation in the drug development process by regulators is now commonplace in Europe and is encouraged by EU directives. For example, in November 1998, the EMEA published its guidance for pharmaceutical companies, which advised them to hold meetings with EMEA staff prior to submission of product licence applications to the centralised procedure. EMEA stressed the importance of this because it enabled companies to get pre-submission advice from the regulators about their product dossiers and helped to ensure that their applications could be validated quickly (Anon 1998v).

We asked our respondents whether the relationship developing between regulators and industry was 'too cosy' for regulatory agencies to maintain an independent public health perspective. Clearly this question is not entirely separate from some of the issues raised by inter-agency competition for industry fees. This is illustrated by the remarks of the head scientist of European procedures at BfArM, who outlined the new goals of the institution to be 'competitive for European procedures, so there is a necessity to provide a system which can interact in a proper way, which gives acceptable results which industry is happy enough with'.[25]

This German regulator believed that competition had made BfArM more 'customer-oriented' towards industry. Although welcoming this development, it was also noted that regulatory agencies should be sufficiently independent from industry fees so that regulator–industry relations could be redefined when necessary:

> Every company is absolutely free to go wherever they want with their new products and if an agency wants to survive, especially a big agency with a lot of highly qualified experts then you must be in a position to convince your customers ... There might always be a danger of being too close to industry. I think it is a continuous exercise to look at how far you can go in any direction. And it is easier if you are not so much dependent on the other side, if you could survive even if there is a company which says we're going to somebody else, then it's much easier to keep your distance.[26]

Thus, one reason for regulatory agencies spending considerable amounts of time offering advice to the industry is to encourage companies to use their national agency for a first assessment, rather than a competitor agency, as this increases the likelihood of them also serving as the Reference Member State. There is certainly a degree of mutual interest generated by the Euro-procedures, as one senior industrial scientist explained:

> You [the manufacturer] want a good rapporteur. A knowledgeable one, one who is on your side and understands your situation. In other words you want them to champion your product. That's what you want and that's what we look for as well.[27]

Predictably, representatives of industry welcome this consultation because, as one put it, 'any procedure which enables an international company to get a drug in more markets more quickly is seen as a positive and an important move'.[28]

In fact, none of our industry sources thought that regulators were 'too close' to industry in a way that had negative connotations for public health (Table 6.3). Just under half denied altogether the idea that there is 'too cosy' a relationship between industry and regulatory agencies:

> It's not true that it's too cosy. If you talk to regulators they will tell you that they are there to protect public health. When the barriers broke down between regulators and industry, which occurred around the mid-1980s, and the MCA was the leading edge in that, communication improved, that's all.[29]

> There's a good relationship because there is a good scientific basis. You've either got good data or not. You won't get by without good data with the regulators.[30]

About the same number of industry respondents acknowledged that their relations with regulators were 'cosy' or 'close', but argued that this improves the quality of regulations and is in the interests of patients:

> I think it is a very good thing to have a good, cosy relationship between industry and regulators so that we are clear about what we actually need to do with the scientific data. I can't see the point in us all working in the dark – it's to nobody's benefit, including patients.[31]

The fact that industry is too close to the regulators is not a bad thing because both parties can understand each other better. That does not mean we will simply adopt each other's viewpoints.[32]

Co-operation will lead to more openness between industry and regulators on scientific issues which will be of ultimate benefit to the patients.[33]

I think that the systems are geared towards trying to license medicines. I think that the MCA believe that if a medicine is safe and effective then a patient should have it, whereas the chief executive of the Irish authorities stood up and basically said their *raison d'être* is to keep unsafe medicines off the market. I thought that was a really negative way of pitching a licensing authority. It should be about getting good medicines on the market, so I believe the MCA has the right attitude to licensing medicines.[34]

Many regulators share this industrial perspective and rebuff suggestions that the Europeanisation of drug regulation has resulted in regulatory authorities becoming so 'close' to industry that they are in danger of being influenced by industrial interests at the expense of protecting public health (Table 6.3). Typically, one MCA official declared:

*Table 6.3*   Industry and regulator views on closeness of industry–regulator relations as a threat to public health ('Industry–regulator relations threaten public health because they are "too close"')

|  | n | No (%) | Yes (%) | Unsure (%) |
|---|---|---|---|---|
| Industry | 27 | 24 (89) | 0 (0) | 3 (11) |
| UK regulators | 2 | 1 (50) | 1 (50) | 0 (0) |
| German regulators | 4 | 2 (50) | 1 (25) | 1 (25) |
| Swedish regulators | 7 | 1 (14) | 1 (14) | 5 (72) |
| EU regulators | 2 | 2 (100) | 0 (0) | 0 (0) |
| Totals | 42 | 30 (71) | 3 (7) | 9 (21) |

Our mission is to protect the public health while at the same time not impeding the development of the British pharmaceutical industry. In other words, it's neutral ... We actually think that by licensing good medicines quickly we are enhancing the health of the UK public.[35]

Similarly, a scientific assessor at the Swedish MPA stated:

I would say we have a very close relationship with industry, and I think a very good relationship with industry ... I think that [adversarial relations] are bad because if we are here to make sure that we get good drugs on the market then we should stop bad ones, and you do so by assessing the applications in the correct way. We should always remember that drug companies have been working, hundreds of people, for ten years on their new drug. They know their product best. We have 210 days, four people trying to assess to see what they've done wrong ... so a good working atmosphere is good for that necessary discussion around that product. And I think also that if we can show that we have qualities and are willing to discuss things, then we can also influence drug development a little bit. Some people say that's naive, but some companies come to us to discuss requirements, and if we can influence the way they develop drugs, perhaps we can also help the development of better drugs.[36]

In other words, these 'pro-consultation' regulators believe that working closely with industry enhances the efficient development and marketing of new drugs. For these regulators, their job is done best by including industrial expertise in a co-operative technical negotiation, rather than encouraging experts to be seen as advocates of particular interests. This also reveals how European regulators rely heavily on industrial expertise, and invest trust in the industry, as they attempt to govern by consent.

Only three regulators expressed concern that excessive consultation with industry can blur the line between being 'independent assessors' entrusted with the task of 'protecting public health', on the one hand, and becoming partners with industry in the drug development business, on the other (Table 6.3). For example, when asked if the relationship between regulators and industry was becoming 'too cosy' as a result of Europeanisation of drug regulation, one senior Swedish regulator responded:

> I give some considerable merit to that statement. I agree that one has to be very careful now. We have this system which really forces you to work more closely with industry than ever before. My experience is that it's a little bit bothersome. But it's the system that has been set up that forces you to have a cosier relationship with industry. We could well do without it … But if you have a close relationship with industry in the development phase, [then] during the evaluation phase, you're bound to be influenced by their arguments in the dialogue and by personal contact … Where you're a rapporteur, if you're going to be successful in the CPMP and further on, you need to have a dialogue, you need to have close contact otherwise the system doesn't work. But also the potential is there that you take too much notice of industry, instead of making your own judgement based on the documentation as it has been presented.[37]

Thus, a few of the regulators we interviewed considered that the Europeanisation of drug regulation is heightening the risk of conflicts of interest during regulatory assessment.

## Secrecy and the impossibility of independent social scientific verification

Evidently there is a division of opinion among our respondents, especially regarding the impacts of European harmonisation on safety standards and of inter-agency competition on safety evaluation. Some believe those impacts will be positive, while others are worried that they will be negative. We wanted to conduct an independent social scientific investigation of some 'case study' drugs within these Euro-systems in order to examine further which of these optimistic or pessimistic perspectives had more merit. However, we were prevented from doing so by the secrecy surrounding the European medicines licensing systems.

We made determined efforts to obtain the required 'case study' data, but with limited success. We requested a list detailing the products, companies concerned and regulatory outcomes for drugs submitted to the decentralised procedure from the EMEA, which is legally bound to record details of all such procedures (European

Commission 1994: 25; Personal Communication 1996a).[38] Nevertheless, the EMEA refused to divulge the information on the grounds of lack of authority. They referred our request to the Mutual Recognition Facilitation Group (MRFG), an 'informal' body consisting of heads of the national regulatory agencies of Member States. However, the MRFG also refused to provide the information requested, as follows:

> information [on mutual recognition products] is treated very much on a 'need to know' basis, and those who need to know are, at the moment, considered to be the applicant [manufacturer], the Reference Member State and the Concerned Member States.
>
> (Personal Communication 1996b)

As regards specific 'case-study' drugs, several candidates were identified and formal requests for access to toxicological and clinical data were made to companies in the UK and Sweden, but all were refused because of industry concerns about confidentiality. The national regulatory authorities in Germany and the UK also refused all access to information about licensing applications because of secrecy laws. The Swedish MPA did provide such information under its Freedom of the Press Act, but only on the rather ill-defined condition that the data were 'not used in a way that the marketing authorisation holder/agent/manufacturer will be damaged' (Personal Communication 1996c).

## Conclusion

The traditional regulatory model of state intervention to regulate market activities is being replaced by one in which industry and regulators are conceptualised as two parties with mutual, or at least overlapping, interests in the drug development process. For some years national regulatory agencies and national trade associations in Europe have met to co-ordinate drug regulatory policy. Since the beginning of the 1990s, such corporatism has become internationalised and deepened as the regulatory agencies and industry trade associations of the US, the EU and Japan have met regularly and become 'co-responsible' for the drawing up of technical guidelines for the clinical and pre-clinical testing of drugs under the auspices of the ICH (D'Arcy and Harron 1992; 1994; 1996; 1998).

The regulatory systems being put in place in the EU further *increase* the influence of drug companies. Indeed, the roles of the Reference Member State and the rapporteur bring industry and regulators closer, at a much lower level of the regulatory process, than ever before. With these arrangements, regulators and companies become virtual 'allies' with respect to an individual product as it progresses through the EU licensing systems. Furthermore, a pre-existing corporate bias is being consolidated by an internal EU market in which national agencies compete with each other for regulatory work provided by drug companies. In effect, this competition puts pressure on the national regulatory agencies to weigh up regulatory checks for safety and efficacy against institutional interests in being the fastest in reviewing and approving drugs.

Whether or not our data suggest that these Europeanisation processes are a threat to safety standards and public health partly depends on interpretation. There is no question that a large majority of our industry sources optimistically welcome the new EU competitive and harmonising processes and believe that they will not compromise safety. Taken at face value, this is significant evidence against extrapolating the thesis of Lexchin and other critics to the emerging systems of EU drug regulation. However, another interpretation is that industry sources welcome these systems precisely because they serve their commercial interests in getting new and more profitable medications on the market more quickly, and that their comments about safety and health are at best wishful thinking and at worst self-serving. For example, in a study comparing the attitudes of 47 industry representatives with 36 academics in medicine towards clinical trials, Blum *et al.* (1986) found that industry's main concern was the reduction of the cost of drug development, even if this implied less-than-ideal clinical trials designs, while academia wanted to reduce the cost of illness by increasing drug safety. Moreover, Hodgkin (1996: 3) has argued that harmonisation within the ICH process is 'strongly biased towards getting new drugs on to the global market as quickly as possible' rather than towards public health and safety.

While the optimistic view finds some support among regulators, the majority of the regulators we interviewed, especially those whose primary affiliation is at the national rather than the EU level, support Lexchin's argument that faster approvals might well undermine safety evaluation. It is significant that the greatest concerns about the impact of harmonisation and fast approvals on safety were shown by the Swedish regulators, who have in the past taken longer to approve drugs because they have imposed tougher standards on manufacturers (Andersson 1992: 70). While not directly linked with greater transparency in government, it may be that the freedom of information in Sweden generates a regulatory culture which is more sensitive to the public interest than the more secretive regulatory systems of Germany and the UK (see Chapter 7).

Nevertheless, half the British and German regulators also thought that harmonisation would entail a 'levelling down' in safety standards. It is important to appreciate that this evidence emanates from government regulators who are not generally outspoken critics of the regulatory systems within which they work. They were senior regulators who would be expected to defend their own policies, rather than express worries about threats to public health to 'outsiders'. Thus, these regulators' concerns about safety seem to us to be a considerable warning that the emerging EU regulatory systems may compromise patient protection. Furthermore, these European regulators are not alone in their assessment of harmonisation. In the context of international harmonisation and proposals that the US Food and Drug Administration (FDA) should 'mutually recognise' foreign approvals, the Public Citizens' Health Research Group conducted a survey of opinion among FDA regulators. They found that 84 per cent of Medical Officers at the FDA opposed such mutual recognition because they believed safety would be compromised (Anon 1992a: 19). Recently, Pearce (1996) has vividly illustrated this by showing that the US was spared two epidemics of asthma mortality by imposing more stringent safety standards than in Europe on the approval of pressurised beta agonist inhalers.

As Garratini has indicated, rapid drug approvals may lead to a proliferation of 'me-too' drugs on the European market. This may have undesirable consequences for public health, because it becomes difficult for doctors to select the medicines that are genuinely the most effective for their patients. The extent of this problem was hinted at by the EMEA initiative in July 1998 to discuss the development of a European Medicines Information Network (MINE). The purpose of MINE would be to provide health professionals with more information about medicines, including advice about prescribing and comparative effectiveness (Anon 1998q). According to the EMEA, such a development fell within its remit 'to protect public health by mobilising the best scientific resources existing within the EU' (Anon 1998o). However, EFPIA objected to the idea and did not attend the first meeting about MINE. The future of the idea in the face of industry opposition is unclear. Other evidence from the US also suggests that increasingly rapid approval times may pose risks to patients. The US General Accounting Office (GAO) reviewed post-approval risks of all the 209 new drugs approved by the FDA between 1976 and 1985 and concluded that 'among drugs approved in fewer than 4 years, those that turned out to have serious post-approval risks had generally been approved by FDA in a shorter time than those without such risks' (General Accounting Office 1990: 4). Unfortunately, it is too early for similar data to be available for the EU centralised and mutual recognition procedures.

A study of the relatively small number of drugs that had been through the Euro-procedures could have provided more substantial independent light on these debates about safety standards and safety evaluation. The consequence of such investigation being blocked by secrecy is that no definitive social scientific analysis of whether the new European licensing systems might lead to a lowering of safety and efficacy standards for EU citizens can be provided. It follows that such an analysis is also denied the wider medical community and, of course, patients. Thus, a situation obtains in which a significant number of regulators have expressed concern that the EU medicines licensing systems which are being put in place might well compromise safety, yet those systems are deficient in their capacity to accommodate independent scrutiny upon which informed policy changes could be based.

# Chapter 7

# Democracy, technocracy and secrecy

While most of us live in countries frequently described as democracies, there are many different conceptualisations of democracy. In Chapter 1, we outlined how political theory could be helpful in developing a framework for investigating regulation. In this chapter, we make no attempt to discuss comprehensively or in depth the variety of contributions within democratic theory. However, it is useful to draw on some theoretical strands which are relevant to the regulation of medicines.

Democracy in its most superficial sense entails the basic conditions of universal suffrage and free elections, but few theorists see it as limited to procedures for choosing governments in which elites compete for mass electoral support. Rather, most democratic theory requires that citizens participate in shaping policies in ways that go beyond merely voting. A key point which separates these theorists is the distinction between representative democracy and participative democracy. The former position, which has much in common with pluralism, advocates that democracy functions by interest groups competing (on a more or less equal playing field) to influence government policy. Governments have to pay attention to these interest groups because they may represent an important electoral reward (Laird 1993). On the other hand, those who advocate participative democracy go further, maintaining that democracy can only function properly if it involves the direct participation of interest groups and citizens in making decisions and policies.

Pluralism assumes that organised groups have fixed interests, which they can articulate correctly, whereas participative democracy allows that citizens' interests may alter as a result of the participation process itself. *Both* types of democracy imply that citizens have access to information about political decisions and policy-making. However, for many decades most governments in Europe have severely limited such information to citizens *in the name of democracy*. This 'secrecy thesis' usually takes one of two forms. It may be argued that the provision of information about matters concerning 'state security' could open the democratic state to attacks from non-democratic forces, thus undermining or possibly even causing the downfall of democracy. In addition, advocates of state secrecy may also argue that citizens should not be provided with information pertaining to government's business with commercial companies, because that might undermine 'fair competition' in private enterprise which, it is argued, is necessary for the proper functioning of democracy (Robertson 1982).

In matters involving scientific and technological expertise, such as medicines regulation, a further challenge to democratic theory is posed, namely technocracy. In its purest form, a technocratic society implies that decision-makers are selected on the basis of their scientific and technical competence rather than by electoral mandate, and that technical experts make political decisions. On the technocratic view, above all, decision-making needs to be rational and efficient rather than determined by 'the will of the majority' or by organised interest groups. Those best placed to make the most rational decisions about technology, it is argued, are those with the appropriate technical training and expertise, while the lay public, whether in organised interest groups or not, are unable to understand the technical problems involved. Moreover, for the naive technocrat, it is preferable that scientists and technical experts make decisions precisely because they are not influenced by interest groups, who might distort their judgement (Fischer 1990).

There are no purely technocratic societies. However, as is clear from previous chapters, technocracy finds some expression in the regulation of technologies, including pharmaceuticals. For example, regulatory agencies are staffed by scientists and advised by expert scientists outside the agency. Together, these scientists reach the substantial recommendations about drug regulatory decisions. Democratic representatives in government are built into the process only in appointing these senior scientists and in approving or rejecting the scientists' recommendations. As government ministers and officials generally approve the recommendations of regulatory agencies and their expert scientists, some might argue that this democracy is no more than a rubber-stamping of technocratic judgements (Collier 1989; Millstone 1986).

Moreover, regulatory agencies and expert scientific advisers often justify withholding information from the lay public by invoking technocratic arguments. For example, until the early 1990s, the British drug regulatory authorities withheld from the general public aggregated data on the spontaneous adverse reaction reports on marketed drugs, on the grounds that lay people and journalists might misinterpret the data. This policy was reversed in the mid-1990s, when such data became available to everyone except lawyers, who were denied access on the grounds that their use might distort the scientific collection of such data in the future because reporting doctors might be concerned about the use of their reports in litigation. However, in the late 1990s, the British drug regulatory authorities were required to release such data to lawyers as well, after a successful appeal procedure by consumer organisations (Anon 1997c; Medawar 1996). Some scientists on expert advisory committees have also argued that lay people have no place on such committees because they could not understand the science involved (Abraham and Sheppard 1997).

Given the pervasive influence of technocratic approaches within democracies when medicines regulation is involved, it is necessary to distinguish between types of information provision by the state and public participation within regulatory decision-making. *Transparency* implies that the regulatory agency has a degree of openness about its business. For example, it may make public the minutes or even full transcripts of its expert advisory committees, and publish data summarising the reasons for approving a new drug. However, such transparency *may* be entirely discretionary on the part of the regulatory agency. *Public rights of access* to government information imply that there is legislation entitling citizens and interest groups to review the affairs of state according to their preference and request. Under these circumstances, the state does not have discretion to choose which information to make public, unless there exists other legislation exempting some government files from release. Similarly, there is an important distinction between the participation of lay people, who are appointed at the discretion of a regulatory agency or government, and the right of interest groups to be represented in regulatory decision-making, by virtue of legislative provision.

## Transparency and public participation in European medicines licensing

Across Europe, the pharmaceutical sector is probably the most secretive, except for the military industrial complex. However, the extent of secrecy varies between countries to some extent. In the UK, the 1911 Official Secrets Act makes it illegal for civil servants, including scientists at the British licensing authority, the MCA, to divulge any documents or operational details of their governmental activities without authorisation. Hence, any information about medicines regulation received by scientific advisors from the scientific secretariat of the MCA cannot be passed on to the public by those advisors without risk of prosecution. This is reinforced in section 118 of the 1968 UK Medicines Act, which requires not only the scientific secretariat of the MCA to treat all information pertaining to product licence applications with utmost secrecy, but also the agency's expert advisory bodies, such as the Committee on Safety of Medicines (CSM). This double blanket of secrecy operates not merely during the licensing process but for all time. As the MCA explained:

> Section 118 of the 1968 Medicines Act lays down that information supplied to the Licensing Authority in connection with an application for granting, and maintenance, of a product licence or clinical trial certificate must be kept in confidence by the Licensing Authority and its advisory bodies. This is intended to protect the commercial secrets of the pharmaceutical industry. But where there is a safety issue the necessary information is given because the need to protect public health takes priority.
>
> (MCA 1993a: 97)

In Germany and France, a similar degree of secrecy surrounds medicines licensing. For example, the German drug regulatory agency, BfArM, does not provide access to information on marketing applications. To emphasise the point, it may be noted that it was not until 1997 that BfArM permitted public access to lists of products and dates showing the granting, renewal, withdrawal, suspension or cancellation of marketing authorisations. While all products were included, the reasons for the agency's decisions remain secret (Anon 1997b).

As Dukes (1996) explains, secrecy also prevails in the Netherlands. Since its inception in 1963, the Dutch regulatory authority, the Committee for Evaluation of Medicines, decided to interpret the country's secrecy legislation broadly. Dutch law required the Committee to observe secrecy about 'whatsoever may become known to it as regards the composition or preparation' of the drugs which were submitted to it for assessment. To protect the commercial interests of manufacturers, and to avoid the work involved in deciding which data should be released to the public, the Committee developed the practice of treating as confidential the entire technical file submitted with an application, including unpublished clinical trials and animal toxicology studies, which rarely reached journals.

Even where there is less secrecy legislation than in France, Germany, the Netherlands or the UK, administrative secrecy can still prevent public access to information about medicines regulation. In Finland, legislation embraces a general principle of openness, stipulating that all official documents are public if not especially declared secret. However, in practice the Finnish drug regulatory agency considers the documentation concerning medicines licensing to contain trade secrets. As the legislation in Finland, especially the Publicity Act, is unclear about the definition of trade secrets, the regulatory agency has the discretion to define it broadly, and does so. Thus, even if citizens manage to access files about drug approvals, they can be prevented from publishing any information they have derived from them (Ollila and Hemminki 1996).

By all accounts, Sweden is the least secretive state in Europe. In legislative terms, the Swedish regulatory agency, the MPA, operates within the context of the two laws governing access to information: the Freedom of the Press (FOTP) Act and the Secrecy Act. The former enshrines a public right of access to all 'official documents', which is not confined to Swedish citizens, while the latter qualifies that right on the grounds of national security and/or individual privacy. The FOTP Act is a constitutional law established in 1766, predating universal suffrage, whereas the Secrecy Act was introduced as recently as 1980.

The FOTP Act places the onus on government agencies to justify why they should not release information, leading to a presumption of openness rather than secrecy. Requests for documents must be dealt with swiftly, and applicants are not required to identify themselves or the reasons for requests, except when a document falls under the 'provisions' of the Secrecy Act. Those provisions, which can permit the withholding of documents, include instances where release of documents would be likely to cause public or private economic damage, or to damage the security of the realm or its relations with a foreign state or international organisation. This leaves the MPA with a substantial amount of discretion to decide whether documents might be withheld because of potential economic damage to a pharmaceutical company. However, any decision to refuse to supply a document is subject to appeal in the Administrative Courts.

Overall, European countries have been, and remain, much more secretive about medicines regulation than the US, where there are a number of general laws on public rights of access to information. Of fundamental importance is the 1967 Freedom of Information Act, which together with the Administrative Procedures Act 1946 and the Federal Advisory Committee Acts of the 1970s permits substantial access to information. The Federal Advisory Act requires that all advisory bodies must publish their aims and objectives and give notice of meeting. As Jasanoff (1990) explains, regulatory agencies in the US must cite extraordinary circumstances in order to justify holding science advisory committees in secret:

> At a formal level, agencies have little or no discretion to insulate the process of review from public scrutiny. The requirements of federal open government laws, as well as each agency's own organic statutes, apply to almost every meeting at which agencies seek advice from a specially charged body.
>
> (Jasanoff 1990: 247)

Unless regulatory agencies can invoke legitimate extraordinary circumstances, they are required to hold an advisory committee meeting in public, and to provide access to the minutes of the meeting, if not a full transcript. The Administrative Procedures Act requires agencies to maintain records of how decisions have been reached, including dissenting views within the agency, while the Freedom of Information Act requires those records to be made public after marketing authorisation decisions have been reached, subject to deletion of trade secret and/or privacy exemptions. However, documents are not withheld or released under these conditions because they might contain trade secrets or confidential information about individuals. Rather, those sections are obliterated when the document is released, leaving discussions about the safety and efficacy of drugs in the public domain. In addition to these extensive public rights of access by European standards, the American drug regulatory agency, the FDA, is obliged by law to be transparent about decisions to approve drugs, by publishing a Summary Basis of Approval (SBA) for each product put on the US market.[1]

Before the Freedom of Information Act in the US, the FDA retained around 90 per cent of records in its files as confidential, releasing only about 10 per cent; this proportion has been reversed, and roughly 90 per cent are now available for disclosure (National Consumer Council 1993: 32). Somewhat paradoxically, it is industry, rather than consumers and patients, which makes the most use of American freedom of information provisions. Thousands of requests for information held by the FDA are made every year, including many from European pharmaceutical companies seeking scientific data on competitors' products. Drug companies make approximately 85 per cent of the requests for disclosure.

Evidently, as the EU's harmonised licensing procedures became more established in 1995, the European Commission, the EMEA and the CPMP had a range of existing models to draw from in constructing their approach to democracy, technocracy and secrecy in medicines regulation. The EU's current approach to releasing information is governed by a 1994 Code of Conduct on public access. Under this Code, access is prohibited if disclosure 'could undermine the protection of commercial and industrial secrecy' or if 'confidentiality [is] requested by the source of the information or required by legislation of the Member State supplying that information' (Anon 1994f). Hence, statutory bans, such as that contained in the UK Medicines Act can be used to refuse access to information at the EU level, if the British regulatory authorities are the source of the information. Furthermore, this general provision allows EU medicines regulatory bodies, such as the CPMP and the EMEA's Management Board, to conduct themselves in secret, and prevents access to data provided by the pharmaceutical industry within the regulatory process.

According to one Commission official, under the mutual recognition procedure Reference Member States are legally free to release information about European assessments, whereas Concerned Member States can do so only with the permission of the Reference Member State.[2] This implies that a product can be approved for sale in Sweden acting as a Concerned Member State through mutual recognition, but Swedish citizens may not be able to access information about the product using the FOTP Act because the Reference Member State may not give consent for the release of such information. Conversely, where Sweden is the Reference Member State it may release European regulatory information about a product for sale in Concerned Member States, even though those Concerned Member States might not welcome such information being available. It further follows from this that the extent of secrecy under the mutual recognition procedure is partly dependent on how often the most secretive Member States operate as Reference Member States.

Some attempts to increase the transparency of European medicines regulation have been made. The most conspicuous is the publication of the European Public Assessment Report (EPAR) for drug products approved under the centralised procedure. The EPAR usually consists of about thirty pages, providing fairly detailed reasons why the CPMP has recommended authorisation of the product, including a summary of scientific discussions about the drug. However, as noted in an editorial in the *Lancet*, 'on specific scientific issues the secrecy of old remains' (Anon 1996a). Moreover, as EPARs are available only under the centralised (and not the mutual recognition) procedure, they are not available for the majority of drugs, namely those that are neither biotechnological nor highly innovative. Indeed, EPARs are not even available for biotechnological or highly innovative drug products that were approved before 1 January 1995. There are no public rights of access to either CPMP meetings or minutes. The declaration of CPMP members' financial interests in pharmaceutical companies cannot even be obtained – European citizens must travel to the EMEA in London where they can inspect, but not copy, the relevant documents (EMEA 1997c: 4).

## The consumerist challenge to secrecy and technocracy

The most frequent and vocal calls for greater democracy in medicines licensing emanate from consumer and public health advocacy organisations. On the whole, these appeals to 'democracy' rest on the pluralist assumption that citizens are best placed to define their own interests so long as they are properly informed, combined with an element of public participation. On this view, the construction of citizens' interests should not be left to technical experts, the medical profession or government officials. For example, Health Action International campaigns for greater openness and consumer representation at the EU level, so that medicines regulation should reflect the Treaty of Maastricht principle that 'transparency of the decision-making process strengthens the democratic nature of institutions and the public's confidence in the administration' (HAI 1992: 2). They argue that 'full availability of information is essential if all parties involved in health care are to participate effectively' (HAI 1996: 7). Similarly, Medawar (1996: 133), the director of Social Audit, asserts that secrecy in drug regulation 'deprives people of the information and understanding they need, individually and collectively, to participate in the planning and realisation of health'.

These consumerist positions are functionalist as well as moralistic. Public rights of access to information and public participation are not only good for democratic citizenship, they are also claimed to deliver better public health outcomes and more effective and efficient regulatory agencies. According to Health Action International, 'secrecy tends to hide evidence of inefficiency, incompetence and inappropriate behaviour, reducing public confidence and trust' (HAI 1992) and 'in a climate of secrecy and mistrust, the public is unlikely to believe even accurate and meticulously prepared official statements – assuming that they cannot be taken at face value and that some relevant information has probably been withheld' (HAI 1996: 8). Put more positively, Medawar (1992b) and the UK National Consumer Council (1993) insist that public disclosure of the basis for regulatory decisions imposes an essential discipline of accountability, which would lead to better decision-making.

The functionalist nature of the consumerist critique of secrecy does not stop at regulatory agencies, but strikes at the heart of technocracy by suggesting that the existing lack of openness undermines medicine itself. Citing the World Health Organisation in support, Medawar (1996: 133, 140) expresses this as follows:

> Secrecy means medicine cannot be honest with itself. It debases relationships in medicine, disfigures science, flaws decision making and handicaps patients ... Medicine can thrive only if conducted within a framework of honest science and decent human and democratic values ... Science and technology

can contribute to the improvement of health standards only if the people themselves become full partners of the health-care providers in safeguarding and promoting health.

Consumer organisations' specifications for the types of information about medicines licensing to which European citizens should have access are highly developed. This was evident from the details of the UK Medicines Information Bill put before the British Parliament in 1993. It was a private member's bill which was launched by the Labour Member of Parliament, Giles Radice, with the backing of the Association of Community Health Councils, the British Medical Association, the Campaign for Freedom of Information, the Consumers' Association, Health Action International, the National Consumer Council and Social Audit (Anon 1992h). In its original Parliamentary form, the bill would have: (a) required the British regulatory authorities to keep an index identifying the drugs subject to licences under the UK Medicines Act; (b) established public rights of access to data on the regulatory basis for approval, revocation or withdrawal of a licence, on CSM advice and on regulatory inspection reports on pharmaceutical plants; and (c) established wider rights of public access to regulatory information about the safety and efficacy of medicines, subject to restrictions designed to protect patients' confidentiality and manufacturers' 'legitimate' trade secrets (Anon 1993c). However, the bill failed to be passed because of opposition from the pharmaceutical industry and lack of support from the UK government (Anon 1993g).

While pursuing a similar campaign for greater public access to information within the EU's medicines licensing procedures, Health Action International and the National Consumer Council have been joined by the Consumers in the European Community Group (CECG) and the International Society of Drug Bulletins (ISDB). The National Consumer Council (1994: 30) developed a six-star hierarchy of information (Table 7.1), arguing that the EMEA and the European Commission should aim to implement a six-star freedom of information policy.

*Table 7.1*    The information hierarchy

| | |
|---|---|
| ****** | Freedom of information type access to full licensing dossier, after 'cleansed' of trade secrets of commercial confidences |
| ***** | Summary evaluation/assessment reports |
| **** | Summary Basis of Approval (SBA) similar to the European Public Assessment Report (EPAR) |
| *** | Data Sheet |
| ** | Summary of Product Characteristics (SPC) |
| * | Patient Information Leaflet (PIL) |

*Source:*    Consumer Council (1994: 30). The permission of the National Consumer Council to reproduce this table is acknowledged.

As regards the cleansing of six-star information, the CECG emphasised that 'consumer organisations must be involved in all discussions on when and how to release sensitive information and must be given the same time to consider the issues as other affected parties' (Consumers in the European Community Group 1993: 3). The ISDB (International Society of Drug Bulletins 1997: 4–5) spelt out in considerable detail the precise types of information that should be made available by EMEA pertaining to the EU procedures as follows:

(a) public assessment reports providing the essential reasons underlying the licensing of a drug and any conditions attached to the licence. Where an agency has not compiled reports for these purposes, its own internal assessment reports must be made available; (b) copies of the pharmacological, toxicological and clinical reports submitted to obtain the approval of a drug and those added to the file subsequently; (c) inspection reports of pharmaceutical plants, subject only to deletion of personal details and materials relating to industrial secrets and individual privacy; (d) adverse drug reaction reports received from health professionals, pharmaceutical manufacturers or other regulatory agencies, subject only to deletion of personal data; (e) the internal evaluation by the relevant regulatory agency of the adverse drug reaction data; (f) reports relevant to the suspension, restriction or withdrawal of drug product licences; and (g) reports of agency meetings, including science advisory committee meetings and hearings.

Consumer organisations have also argued for greater public participation in regulatory decision-making at the EU level. For example, HAI has proposed that there ought to be 'a wider range of organisations to represent a clear public health perspective at the EMEA' and that there should be 'a consumer representative in some of the discussions of the EMEA's scientific committees' (Health Action International 1997: 4). However, these arguments are very underdeveloped compared with the consumerist campaign for public access to information. On public participation, many questions remain unresolved: How is a 'consumer representative' selected? Who chooses such a representative and by what criteria? What level of scientific competence should a 'consumer representative' possess? What level of consumer representation should obtain relative to involvement of professional medical experts in academia, healthcare institutions, regulatory agencies and industry?

## Industry and government perspectives on secrecy

The views of medical scientists and managers in industry, and of regulators, concerning transparency and public participation in European medicines licensing are less obvious and less well known than those of consumer organisations. To investigate their views, we interviewed twenty-eight industrial scientists and regulatory affairs managers from pharmaceutical companies or trade associations, based in Germany, Sweden, the UK and Brussels, and ten regulators from the MCA, the BfArM, the MPA, the EMEA and the Commission. We explored three central issues regarding information on medicines licensing: whether they opposed greater public access than currently exists in Europe as a matter of principle; whether they supported EMEA's initiative to provide EPARs; and whether they would object to much greater public rights of access, such as those that currently obtain in the US.

Of all the regulators interviewed, only one (at BfArM) opposed greater freedom of information in principle. Significantly, over two-thirds of our industry sources did not oppose greater transparency in principle (Table 7.2).

Those from industry who opposed greater openness perceived threats to their companies' commercial interests either from other companies or from the public. For example, one regulatory affairs manager commented:

Table 7.2   Industry and regulator views on greater public access to information about new drugs in principle ('Are you opposed to greater public access to information in principle?')

|  | n | No (%) | Yes (%) | Unclear (%) |
|---|---|---|---|---|
| Industry | 28 | 19 (68) | 6 (21) | 3 (11) |
| Regulators | 10 | 9 (90) | 1 (10) | 0 (0) |
| Totals | 38 | 28 (74) | 7 (18) | 3 (8) |

I would argue that it costs £250 million to bring a new chemical entity to the market over ten years so you need time to recoup your costs. We're a business here to make money, we're not altruistic. That information is gathered at cost. Why should we make that available to a third party without protection? You could seriously affect your investment by talking about a problem openly. Information in the wrong hands can be misused and misinterpreted. And that's the sort of thing some people have been talking about – the right of information wherever you are. I think that's rubbish. What if that information enables a competitor to alter the molecule to make an important product – then that competitor has stolen £10 million of your intellectual property.[3]

Another industrial opponent of greater transparency related the issue directly to her own job security:

I want the company I work in to be successful and I want my wages, so I want it to protect its commercial interests to keep me employed, so I have to say no to greater freedom of information. Data generated of that type is very expensive, so the company that generated it should benefit, not another company.[4]

However, she described her views on transparency as 'old-fashioned'. Our research does indeed suggest that European medical scientists in industry are increasingly questioning their historical opposition to greater openness. As one remarked:

My history, working in [a British pharmaceutical company], was that we worked in an environment where toxicological data was effectively looked upon as industrial property. It was the company's property and no-one else should have access to it. You shouldn't publish it and it shouldn't be available in the public domain. My view is that, nowadays, you can no longer do that. It's already in the public domain. It is already happening in America. So I think the idea of keeping the data confidential and secret is gone.[5]

A very similar picture emerges from responses to EPARs. All the regulators we interviewed supported their publication. While industry sources varied in their responses to EPARs, over two-thirds supported them (Table 7.3). The main trade associations did not oppose the EPAR arrangements so long as 'commercial secrets' were protected.[6]

At the level of regulatory affairs managers in individual companies, we found both suspicion and support for EPARs. One German director of regulatory affairs, who opposed EPARs, commented:

We decided years ago not to publish anything, except some clinical results where we need this publication in a recognised journal for marketing reasons. Normally we don't publish anything. We don't want EPAR to publish more than what is in the public domain.[7]

By contrast, one who supported them from another German company claimed:

I think it ['freedom of information'] helps to improve our development processes, and that is what would save time with the authorities because then they wouldn't have the requests for pre-submission discussions and advice. If you can get the message out of an assessment report, I think that would be a

Table 7.3  Industry and regulator support for European Public Assessment Reports (EPARs) ('Do you support the existence of the EPARs?')

|  | n | No (%) | Yes (%) | Unclear (%) |
|---|---|---|---|---|
| Industry | 28 | 20 (71) | 5 (18) | 3 (11) |
| Regulators | 10 | 10 (100) | 0 (0) | 0 (0) |
| Totals | 38 | 30 (79) | 5 (13) | 3 (8) |

good idea ... although I think, in practice, all the confidential
information has to be left out.[8]

The level of industrial support for EPARs reflected in Table 7.3
may be partly due to the extensive consultation with companies by
EMEA about their contents prior to publication. We found that
many respondents from industry were comfortable with EPARs
because they felt that their company would be able to influence
strongly, if not determine, the information included. A representative of the German trade association BPI, who had considerable
experience of EPARs, recounted that the regulators simply omitted
information from the EPAR at the manufacturer's request:

> It [publication of the EPAR] is working quite good because
> companies are asked, they get a draft of the EPAR, and they
> are asked if it is OK, and what they want to have taken out.
> As I understand it, and I discussed it with some companies, it
> was not a problem for them because all these things which
> they thought could be a problem were taken out.[9]

Although EMEA sources insist that the CPMP decides the
contents of EPARs and can ignore industrial objections, it is not
obvious that regulators are willing to permit such an adversarial
relationship with industry for the sake of public access to information. For example, one MCA official remarked:

> The final say [over the contents of EPARs] is with the regula-
> tory authority, although the regulatory authority would need
> to consider very carefully that if a company had got a diffi-
> culty with something being included, then the regulatory
> authority would need to be much clearer about the basis for
> publishing that, otherwise they could expect trouble.[10]

The reluctance of our industry sources to permit wider rights of
access to information about medicines testing and licensing is
apparent in their responses to whether they would object to US-type
freedom of information policies that went well beyond the publication of EPARs. Just over half of those from industry we interviewed
said that they would object to such policies being introduced in
Europe, while only just over a quarter did not object (Table 7.4).
Such objections are reflected in the industry's perspective on the

potential impact of Sweden's FOTP Act on EU policy. A regulatory affairs director of a German company, who was also active in the European pharmaceutical trade association, confirmed that there was 'much concern' at EFPIA about the entry of Sweden, because of its 'freedom of information' laws, and that in 1995 EFPIA had opposed proposals by the MPA to make more data public. As this respondent put it: 'We in EFPIA are fighting against this publication of know-how'.[11]

As opposition to US-type freedom of information, most industry sources cited concerns about competitors gaining access to commercially valuable data. However, when challenged that the US pharmaceutical industry manages to cope with greater public rights of access to information and that European companies even make use of the US FOIA for their own competitive purposes, some of our respondents from industry acknowledged that they were concerned about the public and consumer organisations knowing 'too much' about their data. For example, one British regulatory affairs director commented:

> I suppose the fear is not so much from industry but from the general public and pressure groups, who I'm not criticising. I think they are right, there have to be checks and balances, and I think they are right to put pressure and ask industry a lot of questions. But we are a high-risk industry and we spend millions developing products. It is a risk, you do not know for sure if you are going to get an approval, you do experiments essentially, and anyone who's been in science knows if those experiments go wrong, then sometimes you have to make the best of a bad job because something didn't work quite right or what have you. And to have someone else pore through that

*Table 7.4*   Industry and regulator views on policies affecting wider public access to information on new drugs ('Would you object to freedom of information policies that went further than EPARs, such as exist under the US Freedom of Information Act (FOIA)?')

|  | n | No (%) | Yes (%) | Unclear (%) |
|---|---|---|---|---|
| Industry | 28 | 8 (28) | 15 (54) | 5 (18) |
| Regulators | 10 | 6 (60) | 2 (20) | 2 (20) |
| Totals | 38 | 14 (37) | 17 (45) | 7 (18) |

and say, but this, but that, but the other, it could be to the industry very very damaging. We employ thousands of people, and we would have to make them redundant, and we contribute significantly to the GNP, and the balance of payments.[12]

Others in industry argued that drug safety issues are too technical for consumers, and so believed that there was no point in such extensive public access to medical risk assessment data.[13] However, a minority of those in industry took a much more positive view of public access to drug testing data. One British toxicologist spoke highly of presentations made by US consumer groups, who are permitted to make representations within the US drug regulatory process during open hearings held by the FDA:

> I have sat in FDA open hearings ... The consumer groups, who are always there, they always make very good positions. They know the data, they know the issues ... If the US position is anything to go by, then I think they offer a point of view which is worth listening to. Sometimes you find yourself agreeing with what they are saying, even though they have come at it from a different point of view.[14]

Furthermore, a substantial number of industrial scientists agreed that greater access to existing drug testing data could be beneficial to medical science. The head of drug safety at a leading Swedish company responded:

> So much data is in the industry and the regulatory agencies that does not come out. So much is duplicated, so much knowledge is lost, not published, [this is] ridiculous. I agree totally, but how to do this? ... it is difficult for confidentiality.[15]

Similarly, the head of toxicology at the UK research laboratory of a Swedish company was comfortable with the extent of freedom of information in the US and suggested:

> If we can actually see that somebody has worked on this class of compound, and they have done certain things for certain reasons, we don't have to go through that learning curve. So if the data is already there, why should we not use it? I can't see in all honesty any real disadvantages ... because if you're

working on a patented compound, a competitor can't commercially exploit the compound anyway ... I think where it is particularly useful is if you are working with a particular class of compound that has a particular toxicology associated with it. Rather than do exhaustive studies to show that it's the same as the one before, why don't we just reference it? It helps you design your studies properly.[16]

That greater freedom of information would advance the science of drug testing is confirmed by the fact that some industrial scientists, who *objected* to greater freedom of information policies, nevertheless acknowledged the advantages for toxicology. For example, a senior scientist at the UK laboratories of a Swedish company commented:

From a commercial point of view you want to keep toxicological data away from competitors. The things you want to keep to yourself are toxicology and metabolism, but the more data that is out there the better for science. It's a problem because if it's helpful to scientists, it's helpful to competitors also.[17]

Also, the head of regulatory affairs in a German company, who used the US FOIA to obtain data on competitors' products, explained:

We use this source of information to influence our planning and development of new chemical entities because we want to avoid mistakes. So we have to get information and then change or revise our clinical masterplan or our ideas about toxicology programmes.[18]

The perspective of many industrial toxicologists is summarised by a manager of regulatory affairs at a British firm, who commented: 'I would see sharing information in the interests of science generally'.[19]

The consensus among the regulators breaks down when it comes to much more extensive public rights of access to information on medicines licensing. The British and EU regulators expressed the most resistance. One MCA official stated categorically that commercially sensitive information, including manufacturing and pre-clinical safety data, is exempt from any openness to the public. When asked what in the MCA's drug product assessment report was exempt from public right of access, he responded:

> Well, everything, I think everything the company sends in, and the company's data as such, the dossiers they send in, we would not simply have open house and let people wander in and have a look at them. That's why we are looking towards something like the EPAR.[20]

This approach may be contrasted sharply with the attitude of Swedish regulators. A senior official at MPA told us: 'The public have an interest to see how authorities handle cases because we are paid by tax money, actually their money, and they [the public] have a right to see how we handle things.'[21]

A senior scientist at the MPA expressed similar sentiments:

> My personal view is that the authorities should be as transparent as possible without harming industrial secrets. Our legal system permits very wide openness and I think our politicians are aware that this is a highly desirable approach and they are fighting against too much secrecy due to EU regulations.[22]

While one German regulator took the view that the summary of product characteristics was sufficient information for the consumer because the consumer 'doesn't understand any more',[23] we found this to be a minority view at BfArM. Indeed, one senior regulator argued entirely the opposite view, that 'we [BfArM] have to bring as much information about products to people as possible, so that they can develop their own opinion of the risk to take a drug or not'.[24] Furthermore, when asked to comment on whether it might be in the interests of the science of drug safety assessment to make public the toxicological data held by regulatory authorities, one senior scientist at BfArM complained that there was too much secrecy in German medicines licensing:

> There is an absolute need for this, but it is very difficult because of legally protected information. Whenever safety questions are concerned regulatory authorities use this information, but legally it is absolutely impossible to put such data

in the public domain, although it would be highly desirable from a public point of view.[25]

Overall, our interviews suggest that there is considerable support among regulators for much greater transparency within EU medicines licensing. The striking discrepancy between the perspectives of industry sources in Tables 7.2 and 7.4 implies that many of them perceive philosophical and/or moral difficulties in defending secrecy about medicines' safety, but are willing to override those difficulties in practice because of commercial and institutional interests. That some representatives of industry fear criticism from consumer organisations is a significant explanation for industrial opposition to extensive public rights of access to data on medicines testing. However, the most common justification for secrecy is the protection of commercial secrets from competing companies.

## Harmonisation towards greater openness: rhetoric and reality

A harmonised European approach faces difficulties due to the very different attitudes of national regulatory agencies, the considerable opposition from industrial interests, and the extent to which regulatory agencies feel a need to appease and protect industrial interests. For example, the especially secretive approach of the MCA revealed in our interviews is consistent with past events within Europe. In 1990 an MCA representative suggested that a court order should be sought in order to prevent publication of the details of CPMP discussions on 'restricted' papers, because of the potential impact of such 'leaks' on pharmaceutical share prices. Reportedly, other EU drug regulatory authorities took the view that industry share prices were not their concern and that the MCA position reflected 'undue sensitivity'. In response to the MCA concerns, the European Commission argued that 'opening up' CPMP discussions to public scrutiny would avoid the problem of selective leaks, and that it was appropriate for meetings of a publicly funded committee charged with the protection of the public to be more transparent (Brown 1990). In 1991 there was more evidence of MCA opposition to increased transparency in EU affairs, when it was reported that 'the Commission is known to be in favour of a more open decision-making process, and most Member

States are relaxed about the issue, but the British have argued against it and the point has not been pushed' (Anon 1991e: 5).

Increasingly, consumers, patients and medical practitioners across Europe have been demanding more comprehensive information about the safety and effectiveness of medicines and, indeed, many other industrial products. In response, the British Conservative Government published a White Paper entitled *Open Government* in 1993. It stated the following general principles:

> Open government is part of an effective democracy. Citizens must have adequate access to the information and analysis on which government business is based. Ministers and public servants have a duty to explain their policies and actions to the public ... The Government believes that people should have the freedom to make their own choices in the important matters which affect their lives. Information is a condition of choice and provides a measure of quality. Even where there is little effective alternative to a public service, information enables citizens to demand the quality of service to deliver high standards. The provision of full, accurate information in plain language about public services, what they cost, who is in charge and what standards they offer is a fundamental principle of the Citizen's Charter.
>
> (CM2290 1993: 1, 7)

These principles would not look out of place in a publication by HAI, the NCC or Social Audit. However, it was also in 1993 that the British government failed to support Radice's Medicines Information Bill, partly because of concerns about the interests of the pharmaceutical industry.

Even before the bill went to Parliament, its supporters had already made efforts to accommodate industry concerns by restricting the disclosure requirements to drug products which had been put on the market, so that drug products which were not approved for marketing or were still under regulatory consideration for approval remained protected by secrecy. The ABPI and the EFPIA contended that the bill would violate companies' intellectual property rights, and insisted that the industry should not be required to pay the administrative costs of the information service entailed via increased licensing fees to the MCA. In any case, argued industry, the new European licensing system under EMEA would provide summary bases of approval for drugs marketed in Europe from 1995. However, as we have mentioned previously, the EMEA's summary bases of approval, known as EPARs, have not been provided for all marketed products – they are accessible only for products approved via the EU's centralised procedure. Most significantly the ABPI warned that if the bill was passed into legislation, then British and other European pharmaceutical companies would avoid using the MCA for initial product licence applications within the EU system, with consequent losses in revenue in licensing fees for the MCA (Anon 1992h; 1993b).

As the bill progressed through Parliament, the UK Department of Health said that it was sympathetic to the aims of the bill, but adopted the industry's concerns. The Under-Secretary of State for Health expressed worries that the bill could have adverse effects on the British pharmaceutical industry. Specifically, he raised as problematic the costs of establishing a more transparent system 'which would add significantly to the fees industry pays to license medicines', and the prospect that such a system would discourage companies from filing product licence applications in the UK (Anon 1993c; Anon 1993f). In an attempt to appease the opposition to the bill from industry and government, Radice further amended it to exclude the clause establishing wider public rights of access to information. In the terms of the NCC, the bill had been demoted from six- to four-star freedom of information (see Table 7.1). Despite this emasculation, industry and government still did not support it by giving it adequate parliamentary time (Anon 1993f). It failed to complete its report stage in the House of Commons, amid allegations that hostile Conservative members of parliament had obstructed it with the blessing of the industry and the government (Anon 1993g).

Nevertheless, regulatory officials within the European Commission, the EMEA and the agencies of Member States have become increasingly aware of the consumerist challenge to secrecy in government, and of the growing support for it among the wider public. In response, the UK government have introduced the Code of Practice on Access to Government Information in 1994. In this context, the MCA began to reconsider its position on some aspects of secrecy and transparency. Significantly, according to one senior official at the MCA, this policy shift may be explained in terms of changing perceptions about public sensitivities, permitting a new interpretation of section 118 of the Medicines Act, which prevents disclosure unless it is the regulatory agency's 'duty to do so' (Medicines Act 1968: 119). Apparently, the MCA started to recognise that public perception of what constitutes 'duty' in the area of access to information has changed, and consequently the regulators changed their interpretation of the Medicines Act:

> We are releasing rather more information than we did in the past. For example, adverse drug reaction data is being made much more available than it was even a couple of years ago ... While we have got to be quite careful because this is sensitive information and companies would obviously be very concerned that genuinely commercially sensitive information shouldn't be revealed, I think as public servants we would regard it these days as part of our public duty to do that. Which is why over the past couple of years we have decided to make our [aggregated] adverse drug reaction data available to other than simply pharmacists and doctors.[26]

This demonstrates the salience of how regulatory agencies *interpret* secrecy legislation, and that that interpretation is open to change by democratic challenge. Indeed, on this reading of the 1968 Medicines Act, *any information* on medicines licensing could have been disclosed to the British public over the last thirty years, provided that the regulatory agency took the view that it was its 'duty to do so' under the Act. However, in reality, the MCA defines its duty to release information very narrowly and 'commercially sensitive information' very broadly.[27] The regulatory agency still refuses public access to information contained in licensing applications and/or internal agency reviews of such applications. Even the release of aggregated adverse drug reaction data was initially refused to lawyers by the MCA until the agency was forced to reverse this policy after a successful appeal by Social Audit (Anon 1997c).

Furthermore, despite the rhetoric of the European Commission and of the EMEA, supporting greater freedom of information, the European procedures for medicines regulation remain opaque to public scrutiny (EMEA 1997c). Under the decentralised procedure, Member States were obliged by EU law to lodge details of mutual recognition applications with the EMEA, such as product name, the Reference Member State and Concerned Member States, submission dates, a copy of the Reference Member State authorisation and the status of any applications submitted to other

Member States (European Commission 1996a: 16). However, in practice, we found it impossible to obtain such basic information. As we noted in Chapter 6, the EMEA refused to divulge it on the grounds that they did not have the authority to release it. Instead, they referred us to the Mutual Recognition Facilitation Group (MRFG), an 'unofficial body' consisting of the heads of national regulatory authorities, whose chairman told us that such information was treated on a 'need to know basis' (Personal Communication 1996a). Apparently those who need to know are considered to be 'the applicant, the Reference Member State and the Concerned Member States', but not the wider medical community, let alone patients and the public (Personal Communication 1996b).

On the other hand, there is some evidence that Sweden's membership of the EU may be influencing the direction of European harmonisation towards greater transparency with knock-on effects for British regulators. The logical inconsistency of publishing EPARs for drug products approved under the centralised procedure but not for the mutual recognition procedure is recognised by some MCA officials. Significantly, one MCA official noted that if it is not agreed by Member States to produce EPARs for all drug products across the EU, then the MPA may act unilaterally, so inducing the MCA to do the same:

> What we [the MCA] are saying is that if we haven't got your agreement, we'll give you [other Member States] every opportunity to come on board with us, but if we don't have it, then we have the option of going it alone. I mean if we don't do it and Sweden does, we will find that Sweden makes our information available. And I don't think we want to be placed in that position. I think we will want to produce it ourselves.[28]

The new Labour Government, elected in the UK in May 1997 with a commitment to introduce a Freedom of Information Act, has added fresh impetus to this trend. Within three months, the MCA was reviewing its Code of Practice on Access to Government Information, declaring that it would make information available 'unless there are sound reasons of public interest for not doing so', while noting that 'commercially confidential information, whose disclosure would harm the competitive position of a third party' was exempt from the Code (Anon 1997h). In October 1997, the EMEA held a meeting on transparency and data disclosure in

European medicines regulation within EU procedures and Member States. During the meeting, in anticipation of forthcoming freedom of information legislation in the UK, Alan Davey of the MCA's European Support Unit argued that there was a need to reconsider the notion of disclosure 'in the course of duty', and that section 118 of the UK Medicines Act 'must not be seen as a straitjacket'. Referring to the possible 'radical change' that new British legislation might bring, he commented that 'we can no longer carry out our work behind closed doors' and suggested that there needed to be EPARs for products approved through the mutual recognition system as well as for those approved via the centralised procedure, despite likely opposition from the pharmaceutical industry (Anon 1997j).

At the same meeting the chairman of the CPMP, Jean-Michel Alexandre, declared that he believed the Committee should be more transparent in order to show that it had 'nothing to hide'. The executive director of EMEA echoed this view, acknowledging that there was resistance to openness in the pharmaceutical sector 'either to protect the regulatory authorities themselves or industry, or sometimes to cover weaknesses in decision taking' (Anon 1997j: 2). He argued that, while transparency needed be reinforced by a legal framework, it was also necessary for there to be change of attitude within the sector.

Significantly, in April 1998 the MCA suggested that a 'lay' person with a scientific background could become a member of the CSM, and sought nominations from interested organisations (Anon 1998d). Previous research had found little support for lay public participation among members of the CSM and other expert advisory committees on medicines. These experts had typically employed technocratic arguments, insisting that technical decisions were involved which the public could not understand. For example, one expert argued:

> The average member of the public expects that medicines will be of benefit, but when these benefits are not delivered as rapidly as expected or with some side effects, then this quickly turns to hostility. There is a constant barrage of suspicion – people don't really understand risk, nor do they understand potential benefits. They don't understand low-level probability and often react strongly to the possibility of side effects.
>
> (cited in Abraham and Sheppard 1997: 149)

Thus, the search for a lay member of the CSM implies some shift in perspective among British regulators about public participation in the risk assessment of medicines, albeit a small one. Moreover, acceptance of lay input into the CSM's advisory process seems to imply that the old technocratic arguments were never sound.

New Labour first published its proposal for a Freedom of Information Act in a White Paper entitled *Your Right to Know* in 1998, followed by a draft Freedom of Information Bill in May 1999. In the White Paper, the Labour Government stated that, under the new legislation, public bodies would have a 'duty' to make available 'the reasons for administrative decisions that affected them', and that, 'unlike previous administrations' they were 'prepared to expose government at all levels' (Anon 1998a: 3). As the bill was launched, the Government asserted: 'For the first time, everyone will have the right of access to information held by bodies across the public sector. This will radically transform the relationship between government and citizens' (Anon 1999d: 4).

There is clear evidence, therefore, of changing perspectives on democracy and transparency in medicines licensing in the UK and at the EU level over the last few years. However, the discourse of 'openness' requires careful scrutiny. Despite the views of some individuals whom we interviewed in industry, the British and European industry associations do not share such a vision of openness. They oppose the release of clinical trial data or results prior to any form of publication, and want individual agreement from companies before any information at all is released concerning licensing applications. The EFPIA also want manufacturers to be informed of who requests information about EPARs (Anon 1997d; 1998c).

This is important, because the regulators' interpretation of greater freedom of information legislation may, in practice, prioritise industrial interests over those of public access to information. For example, following the Swedish approach, the UK Freedom of Information Bill allows for exemptions based on a 'harm test', which could exempt the release of documents deemed commercially confidential and information supplied in confidence to enable internal discussion to take place on a free and frank basis (Anon 1998a). It also proposes:

Those doing business with public authorities have the right to ensure that their confidences are respected. In many cases, public authorities need access to information held by others, which they will only be prepared to release if given an undertaking of confidentiality.

(Anon 1999d: 4)

This suggests that the MCA could have substantial discretion to withhold information about medicines licensing, including internal discussions, evaluations and meetings about drug safety. Moreover, the advice given by the CSM might also remain secret on the grounds that it was given in confidence and that public access could undermine frank discussion. In this regard it is interesting to note that in previous research, one former member of the CSM revealed that frankness might be prevented by openness because of the extensive dependence on industrial funding for research present among the Committee's members:

FORMER MEMBER OF CSM: I think it most important that people on a decision-making body, which is the equivalent of a jury, should make their decision in secret without pressure. Because remember that now a very high proportion of funds for research come from the pharmaceutical industry. It's no good saying that people on the decision-making body mustn't have any contact with the pharmaceutical industry ... So I think the jury [the CSM] must be allowed to discuss in private. Apart from anything else, sometimes you get people 'spilling the beans' in the sense of they are somebody who is a consultant to a pharmaceutical company and declares an interest and leaves the room. The Chairman may say to him, 'Have you got anything to tell us before you leave?' He might say, 'This drug's no bloody use to you at all. What they [the drug company] haven't told you is this, this and this.'

INTERVIEWER: And it is important that that individual feels that he has the freedom to say that – even if not in public?

FORMER MEMBER OF CSM: He couldn't. He'd lose his personal consultancy, his department would lose their large grants, the rest of the pharmaceutical industry would blackball him, you know. It is just as if you're dealing with a powerful criminal gang, you know you've got to protect the jury. Well, in this case, they are not all criminal, but they are a powerful force, the pharmaceutical industry in general, and that means that, if

you want an independent view, you have to protect your jury.
(Quoted in Abraham and Sheppard 1997: 152)

Of the 23 members of the CSM with financial interests in the pharmaceutical industry in 1996, 3 had interests in at least 20 companies, 7 had interests in at least 10 companies, and 20 members had interests in at least 5 companies (MCA 1997).

At the beginning of the twenty-first century, the British regulatory authorities show few *concrete* signs of substantial openness, and there are no rights of public access to assessment reports concerning products approved via the EU's mutual recognition procedure.

## Conclusion

A survey of 23 countries, including 7 EU Member States, shows that secrecy in medicines regulation remains widespread and extensive (Bardelay 1996). However, the extensive provisions of public access to information about drug approvals in the US, where the pharmaceutical industry is extremely prosperous, implies that neither democracy nor the adequate competitive functioning of drug companies is dependent on the high level of secrecy that obtains in Europe. The fact that the US is a member of the global General Agreement on Tariffs and Trade (GATT) demonstrates that European countries could adopt freedom of information policies at least as open as those at the FDA without violating the GATT agreement on trade-related intellectual property rights.

In fact, our research suggests that industry is not perturbed about extended public rights of access solely because of commercial confidentiality and potential infringement of intellectual property rights. Some within industry also cherish secrecy because it protects their work from critical public scrutiny when something in the research and development process goes wrong. The implication of this admission for a technocratic approach to medicines regulation is crushing: it indicates that the problem for industry is that some members of the wider public understand the technical aspects of drug testing *only too well*, rather than that they are too technically illiterate to make sound judgements. Contrary to the technocratic view that the best science is produced when insulated from the public gaze, the implication of this finding is that the quality of drug testing in practice might be improved, because companies would have to raise their standards in the face of public accountability.

Some regulatory affairs managers in industry suggest that greater public rights of access to information about medicines licensing in Europe is superficial and wasteful. This is justified on the functionalist grounds that consumers and patients have no need for information about the safety assessment of medicines because they can trust the regulatory agencies, whose purpose is to protect the public's health. However, the irony of this argument is that, while pharmaceutical companies do not trust each other to respect the integrity of intellectual property, health professionals, patients and the wider public are expected to trust the entire pharmaceutical industry and its regulators. Moreover, the fact that managers and scientists in industry are willing to prioritise their commercial and institutional interests over any moral or philosophical scruples about secrecy is a strong indication that a voluntary industry code of practice on transparency would be an inadequate safeguard for public access to information on medicines licensing.

Perhaps the most impressive evidence in support of the functionalist consumerist challenge to secrecy is that industrial scientists themselves acknowledge that more freedom of information would benefit medical and pharmaceutical science. In particular, some industrial toxicologists accept that secrecy in medicines testing is at the expense of progress in the science of drug safety assessment. It follows from this that a secretive medicines licensing system, such as that which currently exists in the EU, protects the commercial interests of industry and the institutional interests of regulators at the expense of medical science, public health and the adequate provision of information to doctors and patients. The point was illustrated when Dr David Melzer from the Institute of Public Health at the University of Cambridge, writing in the *British Medical Journal*, called for the publication of full clinical trial results before drugs were marketed, ensuring adequate presentation of data so that doctors could judge the size of clinical benefits and risks (Anon 1998b).

On the other hand, in discourse at least, our research suggests considerable support among regulators for much greater transparency within EU medicines licensing. Some of the more recent interpretations of legislation by regulatory agencies imply that regulatory policy is, in part, a function of public acceptance (or non-acceptance) of secrecy. Not only are the old arguments for secrecy and technocracy on the wane, but it would appear that they never had any validity beyond cynical instrumentalism about what the public would put up with from those in political power. Despite the rhetoric, our experience is that the European medicines licensing systems that are being put in place are deficient in their capacity to accommodate independent scrutiny, upon which informed policy development might be based. This implies that current policies and legislation lag behind the informed opinions of individual regulators in government on transparency.

The foregoing analysis suggests that the main reason for the gap between rhetoric and reality is that the regulatory agencies, which are supposed to protect public health over and above the interests of the pharmaceutical industry, share significant common financial and institutional interests with the industry. The EMEA is substantially funded by licensing fees from the industry, and many regulatory agencies of Member States, such as the MCA, are wholly funded by industry fees. Consequently, industry has a strategic voice over whether European regulatory agencies are delivering 'value for money' on industry's criteria, which do not include increased rights of public access to agency files. Similarly, some members of the CPMP have financial interests in pharmaceutical companies, so may not wish those interests to be put in jeopardy as a result of greater transparency.

# Chapter 8

# Conclusions and political implications

According to Vogel (1998: 18), the last decade has seen a change in 'the preferences of government officials' towards medicines regulation, partly driven by 'political pressures for more rapid drug approval'. Our research provides insights into the nature of that 'political pressure': how it was constructed and its implications for regulatory science and social interests. In this chapter, we return to some of the themes outlined in Chapter 1, in the light of our empirical findings, in order to draw out their relevance to the pharmaceutical sector. In addition, we consider some of the political implications of our analysis.

## The European regulatory state

At the national level there is little evidence of pluralist regulatory politics. The pharmaceutical industry is not merely one of many interest groups competing for the attention of regulators. In medicines licensing, as distinct from pricing, the main industrial interests are the research-based pharmaceutical companies. These interests are fairly concentrated, especially in Sweden and the UK. Consequently, there is insufficient competition between interests *within* the industry to generate even 'sponsor pluralism' (Atkinson and Coleman 1985). Rather, in all the three European countries we studied in detail, pharmaceutical product regulation is best characterised by a form of corporatism which Middlemas (1979: 373) terms 'corporate bias', in which pharmaceutical industry interests 'crossed the political threshold and became part of the extended state: a position from which other groups, even if they too held political power, were still excluded'.

Perhaps more surprising are the similarities in the growth of a neo-liberal regulatory state in all three countries since the late 1980s. However, this was not entirely coincidental. To some extent, the moves towards a neo-liberal regulatory state in each country built upon and reinforced one another. Neo-liberalism has not supplanted corporate bias, but it has redefined the interests of the state to be more responsive to, and convergent with, industrial interests: the clearest example being the delivery of faster approval rates in exchange for industry funding of the licensing authorities in Sweden and the UK. Consequently, the regulatory state has less to bargain with and about. The more minimal neo-liberal regulatory state has fewer resources to both develop and police new regulations, so it tends to depend more on an informal atmosphere of trust between regulators and industry. However, there is no evidence of an increase in pluralism as a consequence of this neo-liberalism. In none of these countries has the regulatory state relinquished its exclusive control over medicines regulation to any interest groups outside industry. In this respect, corporate bias remains intact.

Europeanisation of medicines regulation has been growing for over thirty years. In this sense the European regulatory state has been developing and expanding its scope of policy influence. However, the Deloitte and Touche report heralded an 'efficiency regime' of Europeanised regulation, whose objective is to liberalise markets, and to activate the state in the role of enhancing economic performance (Eisner 1993). Thus, as 1995 approached, the European regulatory state brought its own neo-liberal tendencies to the establishment of the EMEA and the binding mutual recognition and centralised procedures. Superficially, such neo-liberalism seems paradoxical because it grew alongside an increasingly strong European regulatory state, but the strength of the supranational regulatory institutions has been gained primarily by a transfer of power from national regulatory agencies, rather than from industry. Indeed, industry welcomes the 'efficiency regime' of the European Commission and the EMEA because it puts pressure on national agencies to conform to the rapid review times laid down in EU regulations. In fact, the 'efficiency regime' of the European regulatory state appears to have accelerated and levelled out drug approval times, to the extent that BfArM is now almost as fast as the MCA. One implication of this may be that Europeanisation is eliminating international differences in the stringency of regulatory standards.

Nevertheless, even in 1995 the more mature European regulatory state was not strong enough to force national agencies to conform to such timetables. Crucially, by then, the national regulatory agencies, including Germany, had already developed a significant neo-liberal agenda. This is illustrated by the remarks of the head scientist of European procedures at BfArM in 1996, who outlined the new goals of the institution to be 'competitive for European procedures, so there is a necessity to provide a system which can interact in a proper way, which gives acceptable results which industry is happy enough with'.[1] The Europeanised licensing procedures accentuated and highlighted key aspects of that agenda, such as the inter-agency competition in Europe for industry licensing fees. Neo-functionalists, such as Haas (1958) and Lindberg (1963), supposed that, as European integration advanced, decision-makers in governments would define their interests according to collective European needs. However, the neo-liberal agenda which has attended the Europeanisation of medicines regulation means that the interests of national regulatory agencies are defined *competitively within* Europe, rather than *collectively for* Europe. Acquiescence in industry's demand for ever faster approvals, along with reduced assessment times brought about by the new regulatory structures and inter-agency competition, are key features of the 'efficiency regime' in Europe.

Grande (1996) argues that the diversity of actors and the complexity of decision-making in the EU policy process corresponds to a pluralistic form of interest intermediation, in which it is virtually impossible for any single interest to secure exclusive access to the relevant supranational governmental officials. However, in the pharmaceutical sector, European government–industry relations have been characterised by substantial 'social closure'. The industry has managed to reproduce at the European level its privileged access to national regulators, while supranational regulatory institutions have offered very limited access and encouragement to other organised interests. Thus, not only are pluralist politics rare: there is little evidence even of *tripartite* neo-corporatism, in which the state encourages 'empowerment' of consumer interests in order to advance regulatory norms of the 'public interest' (Ayres and Braithwaite 1992). It is not that neo-liberalism has eroded pre-existing 'corporate bias', but rather that the latter has been overlaid with a *marketisation* of the regulatory agencies, in which they compete with each other in an internal EU market for regulatory work provided by drug companies. Evidently, this competition puts pressure on the national regulatory agencies to 'sell themselves' as the fastest in reviewing and approving drugs.

As is clear from our discussion in Chapter 4, when mutual recognition is not initially forthcoming, resulting in CPMP arbitration, then the nature of EU policy-making in effect moves away from 'intergovernmental politics' towards 'supranational governance'. Hence, the significance of national regulatory agencies within the European regulatory state is undermined if mutual recognition fails before arbitration. Simultaneously, companies do not want arbitration, due to a failure by Member States to mutually recognise, because it either delays approval or leads to a negative decision on the product concerned, with the existing authorisation in one or more Member States being amended, suspended or even withdrawn completely. In this respect, the corporatist arrangements of the national regulatory agencies have become *bound into the Europeanisation project* of mutual recognition, making pluralist developments even more implausible.

Within the neo-liberal 'corporate bias' of the European regulatory state, both the supranational institutions and the national agencies are keen to make the Europeanised medicines licensing procedures a success. The 'corporate bias' endemic to the European regulatory state in the pharmaceutical sector is evident from the fact that success is defined fundamentally in terms of the industry's participation and support for those licensing procedures. The concomitant desire to nurture greater regulatory trust manifests itself through increased consultation and more social and networking events between regulators and industry.[2] As we explained in Chapters 5 and 6, one reason for regulatory agencies spending considerable amounts of time offering advice to the industry is to encourage companies to use their national agency for a first assessment, rather than a competitor agency, as this increases the likelihood of them also serving as the Reference Member State. Furthermore, the roles of the Reference Member State and the rapporteur bring industry and regulators closer at a much lower level of the regulatory process than ever before. With these arrangements, regulators and companies become virtual 'allies' with respect to an individual product as it progresses through the EU licensing systems.

Writing from a Canadian perspective, Lexchin (1990) characterises this closeness between industry and regulators as 'clientele pluralism' in which the regulatory agency gives up some of its responsibilities to industry. Yet in some ways the new EU procedures for medicines licensing stand 'clientele pluralism' on its head because, via Reference Member State or rapporteur status, they delegate to the regulatory agencies, responsibility for supporting a company's application across Europe – responsibility that would have rested entirely with the company under the traditional route of national applications. The regulatory agencies are, then, 'regulated' by the demands of their 'customers' (drug companies) in the internal market. This, together with the agencies' dependence on industry fees, suggests the emergence of a highly *privatised* form of corporatist regulation within the EU, in which patients' health interests are defined very much within the industry's agenda.

According to Vogel (1998), such practices have eased the process of harmonisation but, as Owen and Braeutigam (1978) make clear, they are also likely to make regulatory agencies much more vulnerable to industrial capture. While such vulnerability is confirmed by some of the regulators studied here, it is probably an overstatement to say that the European regulatory state has been captured by industrial interests, because it retains the ultimate authority in (non-'local') licensing decisions, and has, at times, used its authority to deprive industry of 'anti-European' privileges. For example, industry has not been permitted to choose the (co-)rapporteurs for new drug applications to the centralised procedure (though companies can list preferences), and EU regulatory requirements have put pressure on companies to improve their systems of ADR reporting. Moreover, 'public interest' capture theory gives a poor account of the emergence of Europeanised medicines regulation, because such a large amount of such regulatory activity has been driven by the economic goal of a harmonised single European market, rather than consumer pressure groups.

Furthermore, the interests of the European regulatory state should not be treated as homogeneous and static. Rather, they disaggregate in dynamic ways. The interests of national regulatory agencies in successful Europeanised licensing systems are partly defined by the desire to maintain and expand their national regulatory institutions, whereas the supranational regulatory institutions seek to de-emphasise such national interests. The interplay between these interests is particularly dynamic because there is not necessarily a simple convergence or divergence between national and supranational interests within the European regulatory state. The competitive nature of the Europeanised licensing systems means that the expansion of supranational power and interests may be in the interests of *some* national agencies but in conflict with others. For example, the decision by the CPMP and the EMEA to deny companies the 'right' to choose their rapporteurs for applications to the centralised procedure was not in the interests of the MCA, because the British regulatory agency is the most popular with the industry. However, this development was in the interests of less popular agencies, such as BfArM and the Italian regulatory authority, because they stood to receive more applications than before.

As we noted in the introduction to this book, the nature of the European regulatory state has ramifications beyond the EU. For instance, inter-agency competition has been fostered *between* the EU and other drug regulatory authorities. The EMEA's expedited drug approval process has exacerbated the political pressure on the FDA to do the same, especially as in 1992 the American drug regulatory agency for the first time began to charge industry fees for some of its regulatory work. Between 1987 and 1995, average FDA approval times for new drug applications declined from 33 months to 19 months (Vogel 1998: 15). While much research remains to be done on the globalisation of medicines regulation, these developments at the FDA bear an uncanny resemblance to events within the EU.

## European harmonisation of regulatory science

Unlike the European harmonisation of environmental policies, where the most powerful Member State, Germany, which is heavily influenced by organised 'green interests', has led ever more demanding regulatory standards for industry (Heritier 1997; Vogel 1995), the Europeanisation of medicines licensing has been most heavily influenced by the UK, where the MCA has proved itself able to employ the 'efficiency regime' more effectively than its counterparts in other Member States. In particular, the British flexibility towards regulatory science has been a model for emulation throughout the rest of Europe. This has allowed the official boundaries between 'science' and 'politics' ('non-science') to vary according to the policy context in which they are operating.

Our research confirms the view that decision-making about medicines regulation is not solely a matter of technical science. Rather, medicines regulation also involves social and political judgements. The problem for the European drug regulatory systems is that their official representation is of purely scientific processes. It is on this basis that the delegation of medicines regulation to technical scientists is justified by European governments. However, we have revealed the contradictions of this scientistic representation of European harmonisation. For example, virtually all applications for mutual recognition before 1995 ended in arbitration. According to the pronouncements of the scientists in national regulatory authorities, those disputes were founded on scientific disagreements. After 1995, under the 'efficiency regime', involving the MRFG and binding arbitration, mutual recognition has flourished, with only a small proportion of applications going to arbitration. Yet regulators claim that this absence of dispute is also based on science. This suggests that political changes which are essentially administrative changes (introduction of binding opinions and greater contact between agency officials) under the 'efficiency regime' have indeed brought changes to regulatory science. Evidently, the regulatory science can be harnessed to serve the political economy of Europeanisation.

The influence of institutional and political interests on the Europeanisation of medicines regulation is very much in evidence – some of which may penetrate deeply into regulatory science. In a political context, which we argue is best characterised as neo-liberal corporate bias, scientists in the Member States' regulatory agencies have been willing to alter their science by agreeing to adopt new technical standards for drug testing. According to one commentator, early attempts at mutual recognition across the EU, such as the multi-state procedure, failed because 'Member States still carefully investigated each application rather than relying on the initial State's opinion', and they were 'reluctant to surrender their ability to define and supervise every stage of the approval process due to their concern that this would lead to the approval of unsafe drugs' (Vogel 1998: 4, 17). However, such resistance has been overcome by harmonisation priorities. A national regulatory agency might be 'very loath' to discard a drug test from the regulatory standards, but finds it 'much easier', 'much more comforting' and 'more saleable' if the decision is taken transnationally at the EU level and/or beyond (Abraham and Reed 1998). In short, there is institutional and professional social closure, involving industry and regulators in the joint development of drug testing and pharmacovigilance standards.

Furthermore, the flexibility of this regulatory science goes beyond standard-setting for drug testing and evaluation. It is also applied on a case-by-case basis. Senior regulators meet at the MRFG to negotiate the regulatory science on individual drugs in the hope of avoiding arbitration. Indeed, the scientists who assess new drug applications in European national regulatory agencies meet to develop 'personal relationships' of trust so that 'scientific assessments' can be discussed and reconsidered by phone instead of bureaucratic procedures.

Having said this, it is important to appreciate that neither the encouragement of flexible regulatory science nor the discouragement of bureaucratic relations between regulators is politically or economically directionless. These factors apply in relation to *approving* drugs, but if a Member State regulatory agency plans to reject an application then there is no shortage of *rigid* constraints and bureaucracy. As we have noted, Member States can only fail to mutually recognise an authorisation by the Reference Member State if there are grounds for supposing that the authorisation may present a risk to public health, as defined by just four categories. An authorisation cannot be opposed on the grounds that the drug provides no benefit or therapeutic advantage compared with existing drugs on the market.

Also if a Member State plans to reject a product, then it must inform the firm, the Reference Member State, the Concerned Member States and the CPMP, stating the reasons for its decision and indicating how the gaps in the application might be filled. A compulsory conciliation stage follows within the 90 day period allowed for Member States to recognise the original approval (Deboyser 1996b: 117). This arrangement puts regulators under considerable pressure to quickly adopt a position on the original authorisation, and to assemble evidence in support of their own position if they propose to reject it. These pressures are amplified by the fact that regulators' jobs in many European countries depend on their national agency's success in attracting fees from industry.

Significantly, we found that a substantial number of regulators in Europe are concerned that the 'efficiency regime' of harmonisation combined with inter-agency competition for industry fees will lead to a lowering of safety standards and regulatory rigour. These findings support previous research by Lexchin (1990; 1994) who argues that in Canada a permissive regulatory approach towards the industry encourages agencies to accelerate approval times, which threatens safety. Consequently, he argues that to improve patient protective regulation, it is necessary to 'dilute the influence of the drug companies' (Lexchin 1990: 1257). However, the regulatory systems being put in place in the EU *increase* the influence of drug companies.

To some extent this reflects the technocratic nature of the Europeanisation of medicines regulation, and the definition of 'efficiency' therein. In Chapter 1, we suggested that one feature of technocracy is that the 'means of policy become the ends', and that the political question – production for what? – becomes marginalised. While some regulators worry that the role of agencies to protect public health may be being forgotten, directors of regulatory agencies relentlessly champion how quickly their agencies are approving drugs. Getting drugs approved – a means for providing valuable medicines – has become the end. Regulatory productivity in terms of drug approvals has eclipsed the critical problem for regulatory science in medicine – that is: how can regulatory intervention by governments maximise a supply of new drugs which are genuinely *needed* therapies, as distinct from those which are merely capable of generating profits?

This technocratic element of European medicines regulation is highlighted by the fact that the drive for rapid drug approvals has not been accompanied by the introduction of drug testing required to demonstrate comparative clinical efficacy and/or therapeutic need – in other words, regulatory standards requiring manufacturers to show that their new products offer some therapeutic benefit over and above the medicines already on the market. Indeed, rather than harmonising upwards to regulatory standards based on therapeutic need, quite the reverse has occurred. In 1994, Norway, in anticipation of joining the EU (which did not occur), abolished its therapeutic 'needs clause' in order to harmonise with the EU. A vital tool of regulatory science in the development of a rational medicines policy based on patients' needs has been neglected and discarded in favour of the interests of commercial productivity and trade (Anon 1993m). Similarly, in order to join the 'European club', the Swedish regulatory system has been required to abandon its precautionary 'second-choice' classification of new drug approvals which are no more effective than established products already on the market. That system enabled doctors to be more directly involved in the project of pharmacovigilance, as they could keep track of new drugs more easily. Yet it has been abandoned in Sweden in order to harmonise the EU market, rather than being taken up across the rest of the Union. With the many thousands of medical drugs on the European market, it is sobering to think that the WHO has estimated that only about 250 are needed to meet basic health needs (Dukes 1985: 51).

As we mentioned in Chapter 6, some European regulators are clearly aware of this problem. In November 1997, Professor Silvio Garattini, a member of the CPMP, expressed concern that only 16 per cent of products submitted to the centralised procedure were 'really new', and that more comparative clinical trials showing benefits over existing products should be required by the CPMP and the EMEA. However, at the beginning of the twenty-first century there is no sign of comparative efficacy being introduced into the EU's regulatory systems on therapeutic grounds. In typical technocratic style, only *cost*-effectiveness for health services is being explored as a criterion for comparison between drugs under the auspices of MINE – and even that is in its infancy. While this development *may* be a first step towards comparative efficacy assessments, it remains to be seen how MINE will progress, given the manufacturing industry's stern opposition to its conceptualisation. The EFPIA did not attend the EMEA's meeting in July 1998 when the scope of MINE's operations was discussed for the first time. Reportedly, this was because the industry association believed that 'the value of a product is best determined by market forces', and that 'interference between the doctor and the patient would jeopardise the quality of care' (Anon 1998q).

By limiting comparisons between the effectiveness of drugs solely to cost considerations, regulatory agencies are also likely to come into conflict with medical and health professionals concerned about their patients' welfare – as has already occurred with Viagra. Perhaps of more long-term importance, the regulatory science needed to conduct comparative efficacy analyses in terms of patients' needs is not being developed. It appears that the function of MINE will be limited to providing health professionals with advice about prescribing in relation to comparative effectiveness of drugs, and will not build comparative efficacy analyses into the regulatory science of pre-market drug evaluation. Instead, the technocratic focus on increased production of drug approvals is blinkering the attention of regulatory science. As we noted in Chapter 5, the pressure of rapid regulatory review may undermine what *appears* to be extended peer review under the mutual recognition procedure, because Concerned Member States may not have the time to check thoroughly the evaluation of the Reference Member State, and because of a diminished role for national expert science advisory committees, who have traditionally provided an additional layer of 'external' peer review.

Our findings imply that some expert science advisory committees are likely to become less independent from the national agencies whom they advise, as expert advisers are integrated into specific problem areas of risk-benefit assessment early in the regulatory review process. Europeanisation of medicines regulation is blurring the conventional division between 'internal' scientific assessors and 'external independent' experts. These changes also suggest increased reliance on specialists, rather than on generalists, which may detract from the experts' independence because of over-identification with the drug products under review. It has been argued that, in the US, such over-identification can lead to problems of conflicts of interest because of the greater likelihood of drawing on experts who have built their careers on developing drugs similar to the one being evaluated (Abraham and Sheppard 1998).

While increased technocracy is unlikely to lead to optimal outcomes for public health, we are not suggesting that technocratic efforts and public health are always in contradiction. It is clear that the moves to harmonise pharmacovigilance within Europe and globally are taking a technocratic form. Highly specialised terminology is being developed for the purposes of standardisation, along with sophisticated systems of data collection and management, requiring a high-technology infrastructure. This is a very long way from 'popular epidemiology', but there is evidence that it will require pharmaceutical companies to organise and manage their spontaneous ADR reports more rigorously. This, together with regulators who are more informed about the pharmacovigilance of drug products, may deliver public health benefits, though a lot will depend on how regulatory agencies choose to *interpret* the data available to them.

## Accountability and citizenship in Europe

McGowan and Wallace (1996) argue that shifts in regulatory policy to the European level have opened up opportunities for interests, such as consumer organisations, to impact on the policy process. They believe that supranational bodies have more potential for transparency than the relatively closed circles of national policy-making. While there is some truth in this observation, it should not be overstated. Our research suggests that there is considerable support among regulators for much greater transparency within medicines licensing, but it is important to distinguish the rhetoric from the reality.

The EMEA and the CPMP have produced the EPARs for new products approved by the centralised procedure. In addition, since 1998, the heads of national regulatory agencies have also posted the minutes and brief reports on the activities of the MRFG. Although a significant improvement over the secrecy surrounding medicines regulation in many European countries, such as France, Germany and the UK, EU medicines licensing remains less transparent than national regulation in Sweden.

Nevertheless, compared with the efforts made to accelerate drug approval times, the determination to increase transparency and public rights of access to information within European medicines regulation has been pitiful. The EPARs represent a 'one-off' disclosure under the centralised procedure, whose contents are discussed with manufacturers and determined at the discretion of the EMEA and the CPMP. Citizens have no rights to obtain further follow-up documentation concerning EPARs or other aspects of new drug assessment. No EPARs or equivalent summary bases of approval are accessible to citizens concerning drug products approved via the mutual recognition procedure, and there are no rights of access to information about rejected applications of any kind, even though such information could improve the reflexivity and quality of medicines regulation.

In accordance with the EU Council Regulation 2309/93 of 22 July 1993, a list of the members of the CPMP, together with their interests, must be made available. However, the interests of CPMP members are not published. This list may be consulted on a 'read-only' copy at the EMEA in London. European citizens must travel to London to obtain this information! This situation is even more secretive than in the UK, where the interests of CSM members have been published since 1989. In 1998, three years after its establishment, the EMEA reported that its Management Board had given approval to publish the interests of CPMP members, but by the beginning of the twenty-first century this decision had not been implemented (EMEA 1997d: 4; EMEA 1999g: 16).

Such developments, along with the MCA's recent re-evaluation of what constitutes its duty in terms of transparency, demonstrate the salience of how regulatory agencies *interpret* secrecy legislation. They also suggest that the arguments in favour of secrecy owe much more to the self-interest of economic and political institutions than they do to intellectual coherence. Secrecy is not in place because industrial science, medicine or democracy cannot survive without it. In particular, industry's concerns about greater transparency are not confined to intellectual property rights; they also include a desire to evade critical scrutiny of their precarious science. Rather, secrecy is maintained so long as patients, and the public more generally, accept a regulatory system in which the pharmaceutical industry and regulatory agencies may pursue their institutional interests with minimal accountability. When regulatory agencies defend secrecy they confirm the view expressed by Fischer (1990: 27–9) that they serve as technocrats whose role is to shield elites in industry and government from political pressure from 'below'.

Furthermore, our research suggests that such secrecy undermines the science of drug testing by limiting knowledge flows and accountability. It also prevents systematic social scientific review of drug safety concerns at the level of individual products. Thus, a situation obtains in which a significant number of regulators have expressed concern that the EU medicines licensing systems, which are being put in place, might well compromise safety, yet those systems are deficient in their capacity to accommodate independent scrutiny, upon which informed policy changes could be based. Instead, the public and health professionals must rely on the speculation and bipartite interactions of regulators and industrialists about such matters. The result is that ideas about raising safety standards, which lie outside the industry's agenda, such as the empowerment of public interest groups to participate in 'tripartite' drug regulation (Ayres and Braithwaite 1992: 57–60), or the substantial involvement of healthcare professionals in the regulatory process (Lexchin and Kawachi 1996: 231–2) are neglected within EU policy development.

In brief, public rights of access to information within European medicines regulation are sparse and minimal. As for public participation within the regulatory process or in the construction of regulatory science, it is virtually non-existent. While the CSM's willingness to accept a lay member after years of opposition implies that the 'old' arguments against public participation probably had no validity, the situation in European medicines regulation is very far indeed from the 'citizen science' of Irwin (1995) or the 'popular epidemiology' of Brown (1992). Representatives of patient groups, consumer organisations or public health advocacy groups are not permitted to review drug applications within the regulatory process, and their involvement in the science of clinical drug testing is also very rare. There is no encouragement of such groups in the generation of pharmacovigilance data or even in the discussion of the scientific standards which ought to apply to it. These standards are developed without public participation – standards which then close out data unmediated by the medical profession from the definition of pharmacovigilance data. Even the much less radical proposition that expert advisory committees on European medicines regulation should be held in public, as occurs in the US, has been rejected by the CPMP. Overall, it may be confidently concluded that there has been little public participation in the long-term development of EU medicines regulation, and that those outside the industry–regulator network face formidable difficulties in achieving meaningful involvement.

## Political implications

In order to meet the challenge of corporate bias, technocracy and potential industrial capture, there is a need for European institutions to clarify the constitutional purpose of medicines regulation. The relevant agencies should assert that the purpose of medicines regulation is to protect and promote public health *over and above* the commercial or trade interests of the pharmaceutical industry. Given this purpose, the most urgent and important task is to create a regulatory system which is accountable, so that the public can be confident that it is fulfilling its constitutional objectives.

Previous research has found that secrecy undermines the confidence of the public and health professionals in regulatory authorities (Abraham and Sheppard 1997; Day 1996). This could be a particularly acute problem for the EMEA and the CPMP in view of the diminution of the national expert advisory committees and the underdevelopment of Euro-pharmacovigilance measures to withdraw dangerous drugs within the Union. It make no sense for a regulatory agency, which is supposed to protect public health, to be so secretive that it is impossible for its decisions pertaining to the safety and effectiveness of medicines to be within the scrutiny of the public. It follows that European legislation is required in order to grant citizens comprehensive rights of access to regulatory information about drug quality, safety and effectiveness, barring confidential details about individual patients and genuine company property such as manufacturing techniques. The EMEA should establish a 'freedom of information' service, which would make available on request all regulatory reviews, including dissenting views and the views expressed during MRFG meetings. Transcripts of CPMP meetings, which should be held in public, should also be available on request. The service could be funded by fees from its users, some of whom (non-profit organisations) could be granted fee waivers, as occurs with the FDA in the US.

The possibility of 'popular pharmacovigilance' or the involvement of citizens in reviewing full dossiers for marketing authorisation seems a long way off, if not entirely unrealistic. There is no getting away from the fact that a lot of time, commitment and expertise is needed to review the thousands and thousands of pages contained in a marketing authorisation application. Provided that there are sufficient mechanisms of accountability in place, then that task can be performed by regulatory staff without public participation. However, we propose that the CPMP should have a 'public interest' subcommittee, comprising representatives of patient groups, consumer organisations and public health advocacy groups who have proven themselves to have a special interest in medicines regulation. This 'public interest' subcommittee would advise the CPMP and could also question it about assessments and decisions at public hearings twice a year, not unlike Congressional committees in the US. At least one member of the CPMP should be appointed from the 'public interest' subcommittee. The CPMP would be required to seek, but not abide by, the advice of the 'public interest' committee before approving a NAS or withdrawing a drug from the market.

Given the primary goal to protect public health, it is wasteful and irrational for national regulatory agencies to compete with each other for industry fees. On the other hand, it is important to eliminate inefficient duplication within European medicines regulation. Regulators and industry are attempting to eliminate inefficiencies by harmonising technical standards for assessment across the Union. The logical implication of this argument is that national differences in regulatory science are epiphenomenal to 'good' medicines regulation. That being the case, we suggest that

European medicines regulation moves towards an entirely centralised system. Thus all drug applications would be handled by the EMEA and the CPMP.

Under an entirely centralised system, national regulatory agencies would not compete for Reference Member State status, because it would not exist. National regulatory agencies would be integrated into the EMEA and the CPMP. There would not be any inter-agency competition within the EU to approve drugs quickly. The EMEA and CPMP might be under some competition from the FDA and the Japanese regulatory agency, but as the EU would become the largest market in the world for pharmaceuticals, one can be confident that companies would feel compelled to use the EMEA, irrespective of highly thorough but possibly lengthy evaluation times. Such an arrangement would certainly address the fears of those regulators who believe that inter-agency competition is leading to a lowering of safety standards and a loss of 'independence ' for regulators.

Pharmacovigilance should also become centralised, subject to effective harmonisation of the available databases. The relative neglect of pharmacovigilance within the Europeanisation process means that such harmonisation is some way off. While pharmacovigilance data should be collected centrally, this does not imply that the data should be analysed solely at the aggregate EU level. The national origin of reports should be tagged, so that data can be disaggregated to the national level because of the significant national differences in the nature and rates of doctors' ADR reporting. Until such reporting is fully harmonised, pharmacovigilance data needs to be assessed using national and EU datasets together, when fed into the European regulatory decision-making process.

This development would also place European regulators in a more powerful position with respect to the industry. This could be valuable when introducing regulations (e.g. on transparency or comparative efficacy) unpopular with industry. As we noted in Chapter 3, the ABPI warned that if the Medicines Information Bill was passed into legislation in the early 1990s, then British and other European pharmaceutical companies would avoid using the MCA for initial product licence applications within the EU system, with consequent losses in revenue in licensing fees for the MCA. With a centralised European system, that kind of threat would no longer be possible.

One further advantage of a fully centralised system is that it increases the pool of Europeanised expert science advisors. Taking all the expert scientists in the EU, it must be possible to construct a CPMP in which none of the members have conflicts of interest during their period of service on the Committee. Members of the CPMP could be paid a reasonable wage for their services and the cost passed on to the industry as a whole via 'drug evaluation' fees.

The implication of such centralisation is that decisions to approve a drug or not, and decisions to withdraw a drug or not, on grounds of public health would be taken at the EU level. Clearly, this would involve a greater loss of sovereignty for Member States than currently obtains. However, if the fully centralised system was sufficiently accountable, then it could earn the trust and respect of health professionals, patients and the wider public.

Finally, European medicines regulation should aim to structure the pharmaceutical market so that most, if not all, the new drugs licensed are genuinely needed by patients. This requires the introduction of a 'needs assessment' in the Union's framework of pharmaceutical regulation and trade. More precisely, the European Commission, the EMEA and the CPMP should draw up regulatory standards for comparative efficacy in pre-market drug testing. The development of such standards might take several years and put demands on the time of the EMEA and the CPMP staff. However, that was also true of ICH, which failed to address itself to the harmonisation of drug testing standards for comparative efficacy. We are not the first to make this suggestion. As long ago as the mid-1980s, a WHO-sponsored study of European drug regulation concluded:

> One practical repercussion of such need assessment policies in any shape or form is clearly to render the development of semi-innovative ('me-too') products still less attractive and thereby possibly to provide more encouragement and funding for truly innovative high-risk research.
>
> (Dukes 1985: 91)

Like public rights of access to information, this issue has been neglected by the CPMP and the Commission for decades. Consequently, there is now a need for immediate policy action.

# Appendix

## Organisations at which interviews took place

Staff at the following companies, regulatory authorities and other organisations were interviewed:

Association of the British Pharmaceutical Industry (ABPI); Alcon AB; Apotekbolaget AB; Astra AB; Astra Pharmaceuticals Ltd; Astra Charnwood, UK; Bayer, UK; BEUC, Brussels; Bundesverband der Pharmazeutischen Industrie (BPI), Frankfurt; British Institute for Regulatory Affairs (BIRA); Boehringer Ingelheim Ltd; Boehringer Ingelheim GmbH; Boehringer Mannheim GmbH; BfArM, Berlin; Byk Gulden Lomberg Chemische Fabrik GmbH; Centre for Medicines Research, UK; European Federation of Pharmaceutical Industry Associations (EFPIA); European Commission (DGIII), Pharmaceuticals Unit; European Agency for the Evaluation of Medicinal Products (EMEA), London; Glaxo Wellcome; Hoechst Marion Roussel Ltd; Hoechst AG (Hoechst Marion Roussel), Frankfurt; IMS, France; International Federation of Pharmaceutical Industry Associations (IFPIA), Geneva; Janssen-Cilag Ltd; Janssen Research Foundation, Belgium; Knoll AG; Lakesindustrieforeningen (LIF), Stockholm; Management Forum Ltd, London; Medicines Control Agency (MCA), London; Medical Products Agency (MPA), Uppsala; Merck, Sharpe and Dohme (Europe), Brussels; National Consumer Council (NCC), UK; Organon (UK) Ltd; Organon N.V.; Pharmacia AB (Pharmacia-Upjohn AB); Rhone-Poulenc Rorer Ltd; Roche Products Ltd; Schering AG; Schering-Plough UK; Scrip (PJP Publications Ltd), UK; Stiftung Warentest, Berlin; Swedish Ministry of Social Affairs, Stockholm; Swedish Ministry of Justice, Stockholm; Verband Forschender Arzneimittelherstellar (VFA), Bonn; University of Bremen; University of Koln; UK Permanent Representative to the EU, Brussels; World Health Organisation (WHO) Center for Drug Monitoring, Uppsala; Zeneca Pharmaceuticals.

# Notes

## 1 Science, technology and regulation

1 A new active substance (NAS) is defined as a newly discovered chemical or biological compound which can be patented. This term has replaced the more archaic term 'new chemical entity' (NCE), which was commonly used to define an innovative drug in the literature on pharmaceutical innovation. The more recent term 'NAS' has come into favour because it more easily includes new biologically active substances in an era of emerging new biotechnological drug products. The timing of the introduction of the term 'NAS' is also related to European regulatory purposes. For example, in 1991, the EU expert science advisory body on medicines regulation, the Committee for Proprietary Medicinal Products (CPMP), defined a NAS as one which 'has not previously been approved in a marketing authorisation for a medicinal product in a Member State of the European Community or [after 1992] by the European Community' (Anon 1991c). In this book, we use the term 'NAS' in preference to 'NCE'.

## 2 Opening the black box of European medicines regulation: methodology and terminology

1 One obvious limitation of this design is the absence of one or more southern Member States. Historically, the market for pharmaceuticals is both less developed and less regulated in southern European states, compared to northern Europe. Here again, there are opportunities for further research which could complement our investigations.

2 Due to far-reaching changes embracing both formal ownership and research and commercial operations, it is increasingly difficult to identify companies which operate in global markets by national affiliation, although most commentators, including ourselves, continue to use such terminology. What, for example, do we mean by 'UK industry'? That the principal site of operations is in the UK? That the company is owned by UK shareholders? How should we label, for instance, the outcome of the 1997 merger of Sweden's Pharmacia and the US-based Upjohn Company? Is it correct to describe it as 'Swedish–American', even though its corporate headquarters are, at the time of writing, in England? Does the merger of the highly research-intensive UK company Zeneca with Astra, and the transfer of R and D control to Stockholm, make the company 'Swedish'? At a more practical level, one cannot assume that a company conducts its regulatory activities in its 'home' country. Bayer AG, for example, carries out the bulk of its R and D activities in Germany yet controls its European regulatory affairs from the UK. Similarly, attempts to source data from the UK subsidiary of the US firm Merck (or Merck, Sharpe and Dohme, as it is known in Europe) promptly led

to Brussels, the company's European headquarters. While the categorisation of pharmaceutical companies according to national 'templates' is necessary for reasons of data manageability and methodological order, such use and the assumptions which can flow from it are clearly imperfect.

3 Strictly speaking, from a methodological perspective it may be more accurate to refer to our interviewees as 'informants', rather than 'respondents'.

## 3 National regulation in Europe

1 Interview with UK industry respondent number 6, 6 March 1996.
2 Interviews with UK industry respondents number 13 and 14, 20 June 1995 and 11 March 1996, respectively.
3 Interview with representative of Stiftung Warentest, 11 December 1995.
4 In EU countries, including the UK, there is a general legal provision stipulating that a person may be guilty of negligence if he or she did not act according to the standards of care required under the circumstances. However, strict liability goes further by stipulating that certain groups of people (e.g. drug manufacturers) exposing their fellow citizens to a special risk should be held liable for any injury caused by their hazardous conduct or by their potentially dangerous products. An EU directive stipulates strict liability in Member States, but permits a 'state of the art' defence, which exists in the UK, allowing manufacturers to escape liability for unforeseen adverse effects.
5 Phocomelia is the abnormal development of the limbs, giving a seal-like appearance.
6 Interview with MCA respondent number 1, 11 July 1996.
7 Interview with MCA respondent number 3, 11 July 1996.
8 Interview with MCA respondent number 1, 11 July 1996.
9 Interview with MPA respondent number 4, August 1995.
10 Interview with BOD respondent number 1, 7 February 1996.
11 Under the German constitution, all government agencies must have no less than 50 per cent of government funding.
12 Interview with BfArM respondents numbers 1 and 3, 6 May 1996 and 23 November 1995, respectively.
13 Interview with BfArM respondent number 4, 21 November 1995.

## 4 The Europeanisation of medicines regulation

1 Interview with UK industry respondent number 6, 6 March 1996.
2 Harmonisation attempts have not been restricted to the EU, however. The Nordic Council on Medicines (NLN) was established in 1975 to encourage harmonisation in Norway, Sweden, Denmark and Finland, and there have been agreements between the EU and EFTA also. During the 1980s, EFTA developed a scheme for the exchange of evaluations, with the stated aim of avoiding duplication of effort, and hence market and regulatory costs. The establishment of the European Economic Area (EEA) in 1995 removed more barriers between EU and non-EU states, including the removal of Norway's 'needs' clause. Since 1999, Iceland and Norway have participated in the EMEA. Eastern European countries are increasingly linked to EU harmonisation through CADREAC, with observers attending CPMP working parties' meetings. The latest, and arguably the most important, attempt is the International Conference on Harmonisation (ICH), linking Europe, USA and Japan (Cartwright and Matthews 1991; Lindroos 1996; Jefferys 1992; EMEA 1999g; Cone et al. 1993; D'Arcy and Harron 1992, 1994, 1996, 1998).
3 These requirements were first published in 1989 in five volumes; see European Commission (1989). With revisions, these are essential documents on all aspects of EU medicines harmonisation.
4 The Commission's task in the latter area is laid out in European Commission (1985).
5 All the early Directives have since been amended to take account of subsequent Directives and Regulations. Directive 83/570/EEC, for example, amended the

'framework directives' compelling applicants to submit a draft summary of product characteristics with applications (European Commission 1983). For a review of EU legislation to 1992, see Charlesworth (1992), also Cartwright and Matthews (1991).

6 The UK term 'product licence' was officially displaced by 'marketing authorisation' in 1994.

7 On the other hand, Commission officials point to industry's desire to maintain traditional forms of market segmentation and profit maximisation as one reason for the procedure's failure (interview with European Commission DGIII respondent number 1, 27 March 1996).

8 For some products, i.e. generics, it is possible to use national procedures after 1998 following re-interpretation of Directive 65/65/EEC by the Commission in April 1997 (Anon 1997e: 2).

9 Articles 10, 11 and 12 of Council Directive 75/319/EEC. The procedure itself is covered in Articles 13 and 14 (European Commission 1975b). The intricacies of CPMP arbitration are described in Deboyser (1996a, b).

10 In theory, neither other Member States nor the marketing authorisation holder nor the Commission are informed, but this is viewed by Commission officials as a legislative oversight (Deboyser 1996b: 121).

11 According to the information available on the EMEA website: http://www.eudra.emea.org/

12 Interview with Hoechst respondent, 2 May and 4 June 1996.

13 A positive opinion for Gonal-F (recombinant human follicle stimulating hormone) was adopted by the CPMP in May 1995 and a marketing authorisation issued in October 1995. Marketing authorisations for Rhone-Poulanc Rorer's Taxotere (docetaxel) and Schering AG's Betaferon (interferon beta-1b) followed in November 1995.

14 There were 18 concertation applications pending when the EMEA opened (9 each of List A and List B products). The CPMP also had to deal with 64 pending multi-state applications under the previous rules.

15 Interview with EMEA respondent number 1, 10 July 1996.

16 Since January 1995, the CPMP has normally appointed a co-rapporteur as well as a rapporteur, a practice not common with the concertation procedure.

17 The only exception was in the case of an application for a salt of a marketed product of long standing.

18 Interview with German industry respondent number 1, 3 May 1996.

19 *The Medicines for Human Use (Marketing Authorisations, Pharmacovigilance and Related Matters): Regulations 1994.* Guidance on the Regulations can be found in the MCA publication *MAL 81*, which also details the fate of relevant parts of the 1968 UK Medicines Act.

## 5  The politics of scientific expertise

1 Interview with Swedish industry respondent number 2, 26 February 1996.
2 Interview with BfArM respondent number 4, 21 November 1995.
3 Interview with EMEA respondent number 1, 10 July 1996.
4 Interview with MPA respondent number 7, 27 February 1996.
5 Interview with EMEA respondent number 1, 10 July 1996.
6 Note that Luxembourg has used experts from Germany, the UK and Belgium when rapporteur. But this example is an exception arising from Luxembourg's lack of regulatory experience and practice of 'rubber stamping' other Member States' authorisations.
7 Interview with EMEA respondent number 1, 10 July 1996.
8 Interview with MPA respondent number 7, 27 February 1996.
9 Interview with BfArM respondent number 1, 6 May 1996.
10 Interview with MPA respondent number 6, 2 August 1995.
11 Interview with MCA respondent number 1, 11 July 1996.
12 Interview with EMEA respondent number 1, 10 July 1996.
13 Interview with MCA respondent number 1, 11 July 1996.
14 Interview with BfArM respondent number 1, 6 May 1996.

15 Interview with BfArM respondent number 1, 6 May 1996.
16 Interview with EFPIA respondent number 1, 25 October 1995.
17 Interview with UK industry respondent number 8, 21 March 1996.
18 Interview with UK industry respondent number 14, 20 June 1995.
19 Interview with MCA respondent number 1, 11 July 1996.
20 Interview with MPA respondent number 6, 2 August 1995.
21 Interview with MCA respondent number 1, 11 July 1996.
22 Interview with EMEA respondent number 1, 10 July 1996.
23 Agencies receive considerably less for centralised evaluations than the fee charged for a national evaluation.
24 Interview with BfArM respondent number 1, 6 May 1996. As the source put it: 'Maybe I just use the English phrase – pays the pipers calls the tune – I think it is said. This is also true in our business.'
25 Interview with German industry respondent number 7, 2 May 1996.
26 Interview with MPA respondent number 7, 17 August 1995.
27 Interview with BfArM respondent number 1, 6 May 1996.
28 Interview with BfArM respondent number 1, 6 May 1996.
29 Interview with MCA respondent number 1, 11 July 1996.
30 Interview with MCA respondent number 1, 11 July 1996.
31 Interview with MCA respondent number 2, 11 July 1996.
32 Interview with MPA respondent number 7, 17 August 1995.
33 Interview with MPA respondent number 7, 17 August 1995.
34 Interview with BOD respondent number 1, 7 February 1996.
35 Interview with MPA respondent number 7, 17 August 1995.
36 Interview with MPA respondent number 1, 7 February 1996.
37 Interview with WHO respondent number 1, 15 February 1996.
38 Interview with Commission DGIII respondent number 1, 27 March 1996.
39 Other disputes have involved BfArM, the CPMP and other Member States.

## 6 Competition, harmonisation and public health

1 Interview with EFPIA respondent number 1, 25 October 1995.
2 Interview with German industry respondent number 7, 2 May 1996.
3 Interview with UK industry respondent number 8, 21 March 1996.
4 Interview with BfArM respondent number 2, 8 December 1995.
5 Interview with BfArM respondent number 4, 21 November 1995.
6 Interview with MPA respondent number 2, 7 August 1995.
7 Interview with MCA respondent number 2, 11 July 1996.
8 Interview with MCA respondent number 2, 11 July 1996.
9 Interview with MPA respondent number 3, 1 March 1996.
10 Interview with MPA respondent number 7, 17 August 1995.
11 Interview with MPA respondent number 6, 2 August 1995.
12 Interview with EFPIA respondent number 1, 25 October 1995.
13 Interview with Swedish industry respondent number 2, 26 February 1996.
14 Interview with MCA respondent number 1, 11 July 1996.
15 Interview with BfArM respondent number 1, 6 May 1996.
16 Interview with MCA respondent number 2, 11 July 1996.
17 Interview with MPA respondent number 6, 2 August 1995.
18 Interview with MPA respondent number 6, 2 August 1995.
19 Interview with MPA respondent number 7, 17 August 1995.
20 Interview with MPA respondent number 2, 7 August 1995.
21 Interview with BfArM respondent number 4, 21 November 1995.
22 Interview with BfArM respondent number 1, 6 May 1996.
23 Interview with German industry respondent number 7, 2 May 1996.
24 Interview with BfArM respondent number 4, 21 November 1995.
25 Interview with BfArM respondent number 1, 6 May 1996.
26 Interview with BfArM respondent number 1, 6 May 1996.
27 Interview with UK industry respondent number 10, 12, June 1995.
28 Interview with UK industry respondent number 8, 21 March 1996.
29 Interview with UK industry respondent number 4, 3 July 1996.

30 Interview with UK industry respondent number 10, 26 June 1995.
31 Interview with UK industry respondent number 2, 9 July 1996.
32 Interview with German industry respondent number 2, 7 June 1996.
33 Interview with UK industry respondent number 3, 9 July 1996.
34 Interview with UK industry respondent number 8, 21 March 1996.
35 Interview with MCA respondent number 1, 11 July 1996.
36 Interview with MPA respondent number 6, 2 August 1995.
37 Interview with MPA respondent number 7, 17 August 1995.
38 Interview with EMEA respondent number 1, 10 July 1996.

## 7 Democracy, technocracy and secrecy

1 This has been known as the Disclosure Summary since 1996.
2 Interview with respondent from European Parliament, 27 March 1996.
3 Interview with UK industry respondent number 15, 14 June 1995.
4 Interview with UK industry respondent number 1, 25 July 1995.
5 Interview with UK industry respondent number 2, 9 July 1996.
6 Interviews with representatives of the ABPI, the VFA, the LIF and the EFPIA on 16 May 1995, 30 April 1996, 8 August 1995 and 25 October 1995 respectively.
7 Interview with German industry respondent number 7, 2 May 1996.
8 Interview with German industry respondent number 4, 4 June 1996.
9 Interview with German industry respondent number 9, 30 April 1996.
10 Interview with MCA respondent number 1, 11 July 1996.
11 Interview with German industry respondent number 7, 2 May 1996.
12 Interview with UK industry respondent number 8, 21 March 1996.
13 Interviews with EFPIA respondent number 1, 25 October 1995 and Swedish industry respondent number 3, 26 February 1996.
14 Interview with UK industry respondent number 16, 12 June 1995.
15 Interview with Swedish industry respondent number 3, 26 February 1996.
16 Interview with UK industry respondent number 2, 9 July 1996.
17 Interview with UK industry respondent number 17, 9 July 1996.
18 Interview with German industry respondent number 7, 2 May 1996.
19 Interview with UK industry respondent number 14, 20 June 1995.
20 Interview with MCA respondent number 1, 11 July 1996.
21 Interview with MPA respondent number 2, 7 August 1995.
22 Interview with MPA respondent number 5, 1 August 1995.
23 Interview with BfArM respondent number 3, 23 November 1995.
24 Interview with BfArM respondent number 4, 21 November 1995.
25 Interview with BfArM respondent number 1, 6 May 1996.
26 Interview with MCA respondent number 1, 11 July 1996.
27 Interview with MCA respondent number 1, 11 July 1996.
28 Interview with MCA respondent number 1, 11 July 1996.

## 8 Conclusions and political implications

1 Interview with BfArM respondent number 1, 6 May 1996.
2 As an example of such a 'social event', since 1997, the EMEA and the EFPIA have played football together annually (Anon 1999b).

# Bibliography

ABPI (Association of the British Pharmaceutical Industry) (1963) *Annual Report for 1962–63*. London: ABPI, p. 10, 'Safety testing and clinical trials'.
—— (1971) *ABPI Annual Report 1970–71*. London: ABPI, p. 10, 'The Medicines Act: committees'.
—— (1972) *ABPI Annual Report for 1971–72*. London: ABPI, p. 5, 'Review of the year: Medicines Act 1968'.
—— (1977a) 'Lessons of a decade', *ABPI News*, 164: 6.
—— (1977b) 'Sir Eric calls for restricted release', *ABPI News*, 166: 3.
—— (1981) *ABPI annual report for 1980–81*. London: ABPI, p. 6, 'Medical and scientific affairs'.
—— (1984) 'New ABPI director stresses importance of two-way flow between Medicines Division and industry', *ABPI News*, 198: 3–4.
Abraham, J. (1995) *Science, Politics and the Pharmaceutical Industry: Controversy and Bias in Drug Regulation*. London/New York: UCL/St Martins Press.
Abraham, J. and Charlton, M. (1995) 'Controlling medicines in Europe: the harmonisation of regulatory toxicology assessed', *Science and Public Policy*, 22: 354–62.
Abraham, J. and Reed, T. (1998) *Managing Knowledge and Expertise in Innovative Drug Testing*. Swindon: Economic and Social Research Council.
Abraham, J. and Sheppard, J. (1996) *Conflicting Expertise in British and American Medicines Control*. Swindon: Economic and Social Research Council.
—— (1997) 'Democracy, technocracy and the secret state of medicines control: expert and non-expert perspectives', *Science, Technology and Human Values*, 22: 139–67.
—— (1998) 'International comparative analysis and explanation in medical sociology: demystifying the Halcion anomaly', *Sociology*, 32: 141–62.
Alvarez-Requejo, A. and Porta, M. (1995) 'Pharmacoepidemiology in practice: current status and future trends', *Drug Safety*, 13: 1–7.
Andersson, F. (1992) 'The drug lag issue: the debate seen from an international perspective', *International Journal of Health Services*, 22: 53–72.
Anon (1962a) 'Toxic hazards of new drugs', *Pharmaceutical Journal* (10 February): 112.
Anon (1962b) 'Clinical trials of drugs', *Pharmaceutical Journal* (17 May): 429.
Anon (1962c) 'Ministry of Health: interim advice on testing of new drugs', *Pharmaceutical Journal* (10 November): 450–51.
Anon (1962d) 'Drug toxicity: debate on drug control', *Pharmaceutical Journal* (1 December): 523–4.
Anon (1963a) 'The industry and the Health Service', *Pharmaceutical Journal* (4 May): 417–18.
Anon (1963b) 'Committee on Safety of Drugs: members and terms of reference', *Pharmaceutical Journal* (8 June): 534.
Anon (1963c) 'Committee on Safety of Drugs: assessment of reports to begin on Jan. 1st', *Pharmaceutical Journal* (21 September): 313.
Anon (1963d) 'Committee on Safety of Drugs: memo to manufacturers and importers', *Pharmaceutical Journal* (26 October): 433.

Anon (1966) 'Safety of Drugs: Dunlop Committee second report', *Pharmaceutical Journal* (23 July): 86–7.
Anon (1967) 'Safety of drugs: Committee's annual report', *Pharmaceutical Journal* (15 July): 59–60.
Anon (1968) 'Medicines Bill receives cautious approval', *Pharmaceutical Journal* (24 February): 215–18.
Anon (1976) 'MPs call for official inquiry into Eraldin', *Pharmaceutical Journal*, 217: 427.
Anon (1977) 'Committee on Review of Medicines: testing the golden oldies', *British Medical Journal*, 279: 716.
Anon (1978) 'New proposals on surveillance of drugs', *British Medical Journal*, 280: 588.
Anon (1987a) 'Pan-European regulatory body inevitable, says ABPI', *Scrip*, 1213 (12 June): 1–3.
Anon (1987b) 'UK CSM getting better', *Scrip*, 1213 (12 June): 4.
Anon (1988a) 'UK Meds Division – proposed changes', *Scrip*, 1279 (3 February): 2–5.
Anon (1988b) 'Cunliffe/Evans report to be adopted?' *Scrip*, 1285 (24 February): 2.
Anon (1988c) 'Swedes want SLA changes', *Scrip*, 1285 (24 February): 6.
Anon (1988d) 'ABPI's "Blueprint for Europe"', *Scrip*, 1330 (29 July): 7–8.
Anon (1988e) 'Swedish SLA to get more staff', *Scrip*, 1356 (28 October): 1.
Anon (1988f) 'New UK licence fees proposed', *Scrip*, 1369 (14 December): 1.
Anon (1989a) 'UK revised licensing fee proposals', *Scrip*, 1374/5 (1/6 January): 4.
Anon (1989b) 'Swedish regulatory productivity', *Scrip*, 1385 (10 February): 7.
Anon (1989c) 'BGA and regulatory policy', *Scrip*, 1386 (15 February): 3.
Anon (1989d) 'UK MCA director named', *Scrip*, 1392 (8 March): 4.
Anon (1989e) 'BGA insists on intellectual input', *Scrip*, 1395 (17 March): 8.
Anon (1989f) 'UK licence fee agreed', *Scrip*, 1400 (5 April): 4.
Anon (1989g) 'UK licensing fees debated', *Scrip*, 1405 (21 April): 3.
Anon (1989h) 'BGA shows its teeth', *Scrip*, 1406 (26 April): 1.
Anon (1989i) 'UK MCA sets targets', *Scrip*, 1415 (26 May): 2–3.
Anon (1989j) 'BGA approvals in 1988', *Scrip*, 1432 (26 July): 4.
Anon (1989k) 'BGA overview of delay reasons', *Scrip*, 1435 (4 August): 2.
Anon (1989l) 'BGA must observe time limit', *Scrip*, 1446 (13 September): 3.
Anon (1989m) 'Approval times in Sweden', *Scrip*, 1462 (8 November): 2.
Anon (1989n) '70 per cent increase sought in UK licensing fees', *Scrip*, 1470 (6 December): 1–2.
Anon (1990a) 'Swedish SLA becomes independent from July', *Scrip*, 1526 (27 June): 6.
Anon (1990b) 'Apoteksbolaget reports on Swedish drug information', *Scrip*, 1527 (29 June): 3–4.
Anon (1990c) 'UK MCA fee structure upheld in court', *Scrip* (13 July): 4.
Anon (1990d) 'Products rejected in Sweden in 1989/90', *Scrip*, 1539 (10 August): 5.
Anon (1990e) 'UK MCA director reports on progress', *Scrip*, 1550 (19 September): 2–4.
Anon (1990f) 'Higher fees for UK licences', *Scrip*, 1551 (21 September): 2–3.
Anon (1990g) 'UK a leader in EC medicines control?' *Scrip*, 1563 (2 November): 4.
Anon (1990h) 'MCA's "next steps" into Europe', *Scrip*, 1566 (14 November): 2–4.
Anon (1990i) 'UK MCA explains new business units', *Scrip*, 1567 (16 November): 4–6.
Anon (1990j) 'MCA's first-year accounts', *Scrip*, 1567 (16 November): 7.
Anon (1991a) 'UK licence fees – new proposal soon?' *Scrip*, 1586 (30 January): 5.
Anon (1991b) 'UK licensing officials' interests in pharma firms', *Scrip*, 1594 (1 March): 8–9.
Anon (1991c) 'CPMP defines new active substance', *Scrip*, 1596 (6 March): 2.
Anon (1991d) 'UK MCA meets licensing/financial targets', *Scrip*, 1597 (8 March): 2–3.
Anon (1991e) 'British oppose more CPMP transparency', *Scrip*, 1602 (27 March): 5.
Anon (1991f) 'MCA launched as "Next Steps" agency', *Scrip*, 1635 (19 July): 2–3.
Anon (1991g) 'UK MCA presents accounts', *Scrip*, 1636 (24 July): 3.

Anon (1991h) 'Failure to act case to cost DM 300,000', *Scrip*, 1654 (25 September): 2–3.
Anon (1991i) 'Halcion – regulatory agencies divided?', *Scrip*, 1659 (11 October): 21.
Anon (1991j) 'Halcion discussion in Brussels', *Scrip*, 1661 (18 October): 22.
Anon (1991k) 'Halcion–CPMP sets up working party', *Scrip*, 1662 (23 October): 20.
Anon (1991l) 'Implications of Halcion suspension', *Scrip*, 1665 (1 November): 21.
Anon (1991m) 'MCA stresses quality of management', *Scrip*, 1667 (8 November): 4.
Anon (1991n) 'CPMP confirms Halcion position', *Scrip*, 1678 (18 December): 26.
Anon (1992a) 'FDA MOs oppose reform, says HRG', *Scrip*, 1681/82 (5 January): 19.
Anon (1992b) 'French HM suspends 0.25 mg Halcion', *Scrip*, 1681/82 (5/10 January): 27.
Anon (1992c) 'German public hearing on Halcion', *Scrip*, 1687 (29 January): 20.
Anon (1992d) 'UK MCA turnover almost doubles', *Scrip*, (21 August): 2.
Anon (1992e) 'German positive list "institute"', *Scrip*, 1762 (16 October): 5.
Anon (1992f) 'BGA analyses approval times for EC', *Scrip*, 1767 (3 November): 2.
Anon (1992g) 'UK pitch for European medicines agency', *Scrip*, 1772 (20 November): 4.
Anon (1992h) 'UK Medicines Information Bill launched', *Scrip*, 1778 (11 December): 5.
Anon (1993a) 'Swedish MPA changes its ways', *Scrip*, 1786 (15 January): 4.
Anon (1993b) 'UK Medicines Information Bill clears first hurdle', *Scrip*, 1788 (22 January): 5.
Anon (1993c) 'UK DoH consults on medicines transparency', *Scrip*, 1790 (29 January): 5.
Anon (1993d) 'New EC pharmacovigilance group', *Scrip*, 1790, (29 January): 6.
Anon (1993e) Editorial, *Pharmacology and Drug Safety* (January): 3.
Anon (1993f) 'Radical change to UK Medicines Info Bill', *Scrip*, 1800 (5 March): 5.
Anon (1993g) 'UK Medicines Information Bill blocked', *Scrip*, 1818/19 (7/11 May): 2.
Anon (1993h) 'MCA offers dialogue on future systems', *Scrip*, 1831 (22 June): 2–3.
Anon (1993i) 'UK MCA activities in fiscal 1993', *Scrip*, 1846 (13 August): 5.
Anon (1993j) 'Pharmacovigilance (3) (Report on IMS conference: Pharmacovigilance and the Market: Towards a Closer Relationship)', *Regulatory Affairs Journal*, (August): 646–50.
Anon (1993k) 'More BGA investigations', *Scrip*, 1864 (15 October): 4.
Anon (1993l) 'BGA figures clarify problems', *Scrip*, 1864 (15 October): 5.
Anon (1993m) 'EFTA countries progress with EC Directives', *Scrip*, 1867 (26 October): 6.
Anon (1993n) 'Professor Poggiolini names companies', *Scrip*, 1868 (29 October): 2–3.
Anon (1993o) 'Fact and fiction in FRG blood affair', *Scrip*, 1873 (16 November): 3.
Anon (1994a) 'German BGA – last straw?' *Scrip*, 1896 (11 February): 6.
Anon (1994b) 'German review to mimic UK?' *Scrip*, 1917 (26 April): 4.
Anon (1994c) '26 NCEs launched in Germany in 1993', *Scrip*, 1971 (26 April): 24.
Anon (1994d) '47 NCEs approved in Sweden in 1993', *Scrip*, 1923 (17 May): 31.
Anon (1994e) 'CPMP safety opinions: Ketorolac', *Regulatory Affairs Journal* (June): 484.
Anon (1994f) 'Access to Commission documents', *Regulatory Affairs Journal* (June), p. 481.
Anon (1994g) 'Spain proposes droxicam withdrawal', *Scrip*, 1940 (15 July): 22.
Anon (1994h) 'Germany's recommendation on omeprazole ADRs', *Scrip*, 1943 (26 July): 22.
Anon (1994i) 'Omeprazole iv ADRs – no causal link', *Scrip*, 1944 (29 July): 23.
Anon (1994j) 'Germany removes omeprazole iv bolus', *Scrip*, 1948 (12 August): 21.
Anon (1994k) '*Aznei-telegramm* attacks CPMP', *Scrip*, 1952 (26 August): 4.
Anon (1994l) 'More changes at German agency?' *Scrip*, 1978 (25 November): 5.
Anon (1994m) 'EC future systems legislation', *Regulatory Affairs Journal* (November): 968–70.
Anon (1994n) 'Sweden's MPA alters approval policy', *Scrip*, 1980 (2 December): 7.
Anon (1995a) 'German officials and management style', *Scrip*, 1990 (13 January): 6.

Anon (1995b) 'LIF and RUFI merge in Sweden', *Scrip*, 1995 (31 January): 2.
Anon (1995c) 'German review concerns', *Scrip*, 2028 (26 May): 3.
Anon (1995d) 'EMEA update', *Regulatory Affairs Journal* (September): 764.
Anon (1995e) 'Update on EU so far', *Scrip*, 2071 (24 October): 4
Anon (1995f) 'Swedish NCEs in 1994/95', *Scrip*, 2073 (31 October): 27.
Anon (1995g) 'The role of the Swedish MPA within the new EC regulatory frame-work' (transcript of interview with K. Strandberg and Tomas Lonngren by the editor), *Regulatory Affairs Journal* (December): 1005–9.
Anon (1995h) 'Oral contraceptives and thrombo-embolism', *Regulatory Affairs Journal* (December): 1066–8.
Anon (1996a) 'Euromedicines evaluation: the striptease begins', *Lancet*, 347 (24 February): 483.
Anon (1996b) 'Problems with three EU approvals', *Scrip*, 2109 (8 March): 20.
Anon (1996c) 'The EMEA – One Year On (2)' (interview with F. Sauer by R.J. Harman), *Regulatory Affairs Journal* (March): 177–81.
Anon (1996d) 'Innovative Medicinal Products: SOP scientific advice to be given by the CPMP', *Regulatory Affairs Journal* (June): 492–4.
Anon (1996e) 'Secrets about drugs are not healthy', *Lancet*, 384 (21 September): 765.
Anon (1996f) 'Contentious areas in mutual recognition', *Scrip*, 2190 (17 December): 4.
Anon (1997a) 'EMEA could go to EC consumer DG', *Scrip*, 2201 (28 January): 6.
Anon (1997b) 'BfArM opens product database to public', *Scrip*, 2206 (14 February): 7.
Anon (1997c) 'UK gives lawyers access to ADR data', *Scrip*, 2212 (7 March): 3.
Anon (1997d) 'Poor response on EMEA transparency', *Scrip*, 2237 (3 June): 2.
Anon (1997e) 'Mutual recognition back to basics', *Scrip*, 2238 (6 June): 5.
Anon (1997f) 'End in sight for EU/US mutual recognition deal?' *Scrip*, 2240 (13 June): 5.
Anon (1997g) 'EC mutual recognition fading fast', *Scrip*, 2254 (1 August): 4.
Anon (1997h) 'UK MCA's revised guidance on access', *Scrip*, 2260 (22 August): 3.
Anon (1997i) 'Pharmacovigilance – second line of UK defence', *Scrip*, 2278 (24 October): 6.
Anon (1997j) 'Shift towards more data disclosure in EC', *Scrip*, 2283 (11 November): 2.
Anon (1997k) 'EC Commission's pharma plans', *Scrip*, 2286 (21 November): 3.
Anon (1997l) 'Too many "me-toos" in EC', *Scrip*, 2287 (25 November): 2.
Anon (1997m) 'EFPIA gives details of new structure', *Scrip*, 2288 (28 November): 3.
Anon (1997n) 'Oral contraceptives off the hook in Germany', *Scrip*, 2296/97 (26/30 December): 2.
Anon (1998a) 'UK may be forced to justify licensing decisions', *Scrip*, 2300 (14 January): 3.
Anon (1998b) 'UK call for full clinical trial results', *Scrip*, 2317 (13 March): 4.
Anon (1998c) 'ABPI responds on UK FOI White Paper', *Scrip*, 2321 (27 March): 4.
Anon (1998d) ' "Lay" member of UK CSM possible', *Scrip*, 2330 (29 April): 3.
Anon (1998e) 'Viagra breaks all records in the US', *Scrip*, 2331 (1 May): 20.
Anon (1998f) 'EC pharmacovigilance guidelines soon', *Scrip*, 2337 (22 May): 5.
Anon (1998g) 'EFPIA vision of regulation post-2000', *Scrip*, 2338/39 (27/29 May): 4.
Anon (1998h) 'Opthalmologists warn of Viagra visual problems', *Scrip*, 2338/39 (27/29 May): 23.
Anon (1998i) 'Viagra recommended for EC approval', *Scrip*, 2338/39 (27/29 May): 36.
Anon (1998j) 'Growing demand for Viagra in Europe', *Scrip*, 2340 (3 June): 4.
Anon (1998k) 'New break-out procedure for MR', *Scrip*, 2349 (3 July): 3.
Anon (1998l) 'Pfizer responds to Viagra safety concerns', *Scrip*, 2350 (8 July): 24.
Anon (1998m) 'US insurers turn down Viagra citing lack of safety data', *Scrip*, 2351 (10 July): 14.
Anon (1998n) 'No Viagra reimbursement in EU?' *Scrip*, 2351 (10 July): 3.
Anon (1998o) 'Will EC's MINE make UK's NICE redundant?' *Scrip*, 2352 (15 July): 5.
Anon (1998p) 'FDA cites more deaths in Viagra users', *Scrip*, 2355 (24 July): 17.
Anon (1998q) 'MINE for information', *Scrip*, 2357 (31 July): 4.

Anon (1998r) 'UK MCA reviews its year', *Scrip*, 2357 (31 July): 5.
Anon (1998s) 'German pharmacy market in 1997', *Scrip*, 2365 (28 August): 3.
Anon (1998t) 'UK ADR reports declining', *Scrip*, 2369 (11 September): 5.
Anon (1998u) 'Viagra roll-out in Europe', *Scrip*, 2381 (23 October): 5.
Anon (1998v) 'EMEA's pre-submission guidance', *Scrip*, 2391 (27 November): 2.
Anon (1998w) 'MCA wants £27 million fee income', *Scrip* (16 December): 2.
Anon (1999a) 'No flexibility in UK NICE advice', *Scrip*, 2439 (21 May): 6.
Anon (1999b) 'EC Commission boosts approvals', *Scrip*, 2441 (28 May): 2.
Anon (1999c) 'UK rules DoH Viagra circular unlawful', *Scrip*, 2441 (28 May): 4.
Anon (1999d) 'UK bill to increase transparency?' *Scrip*, 2441 (28 May): 4.
Apoteksbolaget (1994) *Annual report for 1994*. Stockholm: Apoteksbolaget.
Astra AB (1995) *Annual Report for 1994*. Gartuna: Astra.
Atkinson, M.M. and Coleman, W.D. (1985) 'Corporatism and industrial policy' in
    A. Cawson (ed.) *Organised Interests and the State*. London: Sage, pp. 22–44.
Ayres, I. and Braithwaite, J. (1992) *Responsive Regulation: Transcending the
    Deregulation Debate*. Oxford: Oxford University Press.
Bardelay, D. (1996) 'An ISDB survey to assess the degree of transparency of drug
    regulatory agencies', *International Journal of Risk and Safety in Medicine*, 9:
    151–5.
Barnes, B. (1985) *About Science*. Oxford: Basil Blackwell.
Barnes, J.M. and Denz, F.A. (1954) 'Experimental methods used in determining
    chronic toxicity: a critical review', *Pharmacological Reviews*, 6: 191–242.
Barrowcliffe, S. (1996) 'Developing a global strategy', *Drug Information Journal*,
    28: 523–31.
Beck, U. (1992) *Risk Society: Towards a New Modernity*. London: Sage.
Begg, I. (1996) 'Regulation in the European Union', *Journal of European Public
    Policy*, 3: 526–35.
Bernstein, M. (1955) *Regulating Business by Independent Commission*. New
    Jersey: Princeton University Press.
Binns, T.B. (1980) 'The Committee on Review of Medicines', *British Medical
    Journal*, 281: 1614–15.
Blum, A.L., Chalmers, T.E., Deutsch, E., Koch-Wess, J., Langman, M., Rosen, A.,
    Tygstrup, N. and Zentgraf, R. (1986) 'Differing attitudes of industry and
    academia towards controlled clinical trials', *European Journal of Clinical Inves-
    tigation*, 16: 455–60.
Boehmer-Christiansen, S. and Skea, J. (1991) *Acid Politics: Environmental and
    Energy Policies in Britain and Germany*. London: Belhaven Press.
Boreus, K. (1997) 'The shift to the right: neo-liberalism in argumentation and
    language in the Swedish public debate since 1969', *European Journal of Polit-
    ical Research*, 31: 257–86.
Bottiger, L.E. (1988) 'The Swedish medicines regulatory system – with some notes
    on the Scandinavia situation' in S.R. Walker and J.R. Griffin (eds) *International
    Medicines Regulation – A Look Forward to 1992*. Dordrecht/Boston/London:
    Kluwer Academic Publishers, pp. 111–15.
Braithwaite, J. (1986) *Corporate Crime in the Pharmaceutical Industry*. London:
    Routledge and Kegan Paul.
Breggin, P. (1993) *Toxic Psychiatry: Drugs and Electronic Therapy: The Truth and
    the Better Alternatives*. London: HarperCollins.
Brickman, R., Jasanoff, S. and Ilgen, T. (1985) *Controlling Chemicals: The Politics of
    Regulation in Europe and the United States*. Ithaca, NY: Cornell University Press.
Brown, P. (1987) 'Popular epidemiology: community response to toxic waste
    induced disease in Woburn, Massachusetts', *Science, Technology and Human
    Values*, 12: 78–85.
—— (1990) 'EC unease over UK MCA approach', *Scrip*, 1564 (7 November): 9.
—— (1992) 'Popular epidemiology and toxic waste contamination', *Journal of
    Health and Social Behaviour*, 33: 267–81.
Brown, V.K. (1988) *Acute and Sub-acute Toxicology*. London: Edward Arnold.
Burley, D.M. and Glynne, A. (1985) 'Clinical trials' in D.M. Burley and T.B. Binns
    (eds) *Pharmaceutical medicine*. London: Edward Arnold.
Burson Marsteller (1994) *Results of an Attitude Inquiry Commissioned by the
    Swedish Medical Products Agency*, 21 April. Stockholm: Burson Marsteller.

230    Bibliography

—— (1995) *Final Report on Attitude Survey for the Swedish Medical Products Agency*, 8 December. Stockholm: Burson Marsteller.
Burstall, M.L. (1990) *1992 and the Pharmaceutical Industry*. London: Institute of Economic Affairs, Health and Welfare Unit.
Cartwright, A.C. and Matthews, B.R. (eds) (1991) *Pharmaceutical Product Licensing: Requirements for Europe*. Chichester: Ellis Harwood.
Carvalho de Mello, J.M. and Machado de Freitas, C. (1998) 'Social interests, contextualisation and uncertainties in risk assessment', *Social Studies of Science*, 28: 401–21.
Cawson, A. (1986) *Corporatism and Political Theory*. Oxford: Basil Blackwell.
Cecchini, P. (1988) *The European Challenge, 1992*. Aldershot, England: Wildwood House.
Charlesworth, F. (1992) 'Guide to the European Directives concerning medicines' in J. P. Griffin (ed.) *Medicines: Regulation, Risk and Research*. Belfast: Queen's University Press.
Chetley, A. (1990) *A Healthy Business? World Health and the Pharmaceutical Industry*. London: Zed Books.
—— (1995) *Problem Drugs*. London: Zed Books.
CIOMS (Council for the International Organisation of Medicines) (1990) *CIOMS Working Group Final Report: International Reporting of Adverse Drug Reactions*. Geneva: CIOMS.
—— (1992) *CIOMS Working Group Final Report: International Reporting of Periodic Drug Safety Update Summaries*. Geneva: CIOMS.
CM 2290 (1993) *Open Government*. London: HMSO.
Cmnd 3395 (1967) *Forthcoming Legislation on the Safety, Quality and Description of Drugs and Medicines*. London: HMSO.
Collier, J. (1985) 'Licensing and provision of medicines in the UK: an appraisal', *Lancet* (17 August): 377–80.
—— (1989) *The Health Conspiracy*. London: Century.
Cone, M., Couper, M.R., Dunne, J.F. and Thomas, M. (1992) 'Harmonisation of international registration requirements for pharmaceuticals' in J.P. Griffin (ed.) *Medicines: Regulation, Research and Risk*. Belfast: Queen's University Press.
Cone, M., D'Arcy, P.F. and Harron, D.W.G. (1993) 'Harmonisation of international registration requirements for pharmaceuticals' in J.P. Griffin (ed.) *Medicines: Regulation, Research, and Risk*. Belfast: Queen's University Press.
Consumers in the European Community Group (1993) *Access to Information in the EU: Summary and Recommendations*. London: CECG.
Contrera, J.F., Degeorge, J. and Jacobs, A.C. (1993) 'A retrospective comparison of the results of 6 and 12 month non-rodent toxicity studies', *Adverse Drug Reaction Toxicology Review*, 12: 63–76.
CPMP (Committee for Proprietary Medicinal Products) (1989) *Pharmacovigilance in the framework of CPMP activities (III/823/89)*.
—— (1990) *A rapid alert system (III/3917/90)*.
—— (1991a) *Procedure for exchanging information (III/3366/91)*.
—— (1991b) *Procedure on causality clarification (III/3445/91)*.
Cromie, B.J. (1980) 'Testing new drugs in the UK', *Journal of the Royal Society of Medicine*, 73: 379–80.
CSD (Committee on Safety of Drugs) (1972) *Report for Year Ending 1971*. London: HMSO.
CSM (Committee on Safety of Medicines) (1978) *Annual Report for 1977*. London: HMSO.
—— (1996) *Annual Reports for 1995: Medicines Act 1968 Advisory Bodies*. London: HMSO.
Daemmrich, A. (2000) 'Regulatory laws and political culture in the US and Germany' in J. Abraham, A. Twose and H. Lawton-Smith (eds) *Regulation of the Pharmaceutical Industry*. London: Macmillan.
Darbourne, A. (1995) 'ADR monitoring – towards a better system', *Scrip Magazine* (May): 34–8.
D'Arcy, P.F. and Harron, D.W.G. (eds) (1992) *Proceedings of the First International Conference on Harmonisation, Brussels 1991*. Belfast: Queen's University, Belfast.

—— (1994) *Proceedings of the Second International Conference on Harmonisation, Orlando 1993*. Belfast: Queen's University, Belfast.
—— (eds) (1996) *Proceedings of the Third International Conference on Harmonisation, Yokohama 1995*. Belfast: Queen's University, Belfast.
—— (1998) *Proceedings of the Fourth International Conference on Harmonisation, Brussels 1997*. Belfast: Greystone Books.
Davies, J. (1994) 'Regulatory focus on Europe. Part iv. The Nordic countries: Norway, Sweden, Finland and Denmark', *BIRA Journal*, 13: 16–22.
Davis, P. (1997) *Managing Medicines: Public Policy and Therapeutic Drugs*. Buckingham: Open University Press.
Day, M. (1996) 'Secrecy destroys faith in drug safety', *New Scientist* (28 September): 4.
—— (1996) 'US drug safety regime flawed', *New Scientist* (9 November): 7.
Deboyser, P. (1996a) 'New EC procedures for authorisation of medicinal products (1)', *Regulatory Affairs Journal* (January): 6–15.
—— (1996b) 'New EC procedures for authorisation of medicinal products (2)', *Regulatory Affairs Journal* (February): 111–21.
Delamothe, T. (1989) 'Drug watchdogs and the drug industry', *British Medical Journal*, 299: 476.
Department of Health (1971) *Safety of Drugs, Final Report of the Joint Sub-Committee of the Standing Medical Advisory Committees*. London: HMSO.
Department of Health and Social Security (DHSS) (1981) *MLX 130 Medicines Act 1968: Data Requirements for Clinical Trial Certificates*. London: DHSS.
Dower, M. (1995) 'The EMEA – front door to Europe', *Scrip Magazine* (March): 49–52.
Dukes, M.N.G. (1985) *The Effects of Drug Regulation: A Survey Based on the European Studies of Drug Regulation*. Lancaster: MTP Press.
—— (1996) 'Drug regulation and the tradition of secrecy', *International Journal of Risk and Safety in Medicine*, 9: 143–50.
Edgar, H. and Rothman, D.J. (1990) 'New rules for new drugs: the challenge of AIDS to the regulatory process', *The Milbank Quarterly*, 68 (Suppl. 1): 111–42.
Eisner, M.A. (1993) *Regulatory Politics in Transition*. Baltimore: Johns Hopkins University Press.
EMEA (European Agency for the Evaluation of Medicinal Products) (1995a) 'Position statement of the CPMP on oral contraceptives containing Gestodene and Desogestrel', CPMP/PhV/696/95 (27 October 1995).
—— (1995b) Press release, 27 October.
—— (1996a) *EMEA Directory*, 12 January.
—— (1996b) 'Scientific advice to be given by the CPMP for innovative medicinal products' (15 February).
—— (1996c) Electronic message from E. Koskinen to G. Lewis, 14 May.
—— (1996d) *Standing Operating Procedure (SOP), Arbitration under the Decentralised Procedure for Marketing Authorisations*. EMEA: London.
—— (1996e) *General Report on the Activities of the European Medicines Evaluation Agency 1995*. EMEA: London.
—— (1997a) 'Position statement of the CPMP on oral contraceptives containing Gestodene and Desogestrel', CPMP/173/97 Rev. 2 (22 January).
—— (1997b) 'Conduct of pharmacovigilance for centrally authorised products', CPMP/183/97 (15 April).
—— (1997c) 'Interim report on the consultation exercise on transparency and access to documents at the EMEA', 28 April.
—— (1997d) 'Decision on access to documents of the EMEA', 3 December (no document number).
—— (1998a) 'Principles of providing the World Health Organisation with pharmacovigilance information', CPMP/PhVWP/053/98 (19 January).
—— (1998b) 'Position paper on voting in the framework of the discussion and adoption of CPMP opinions', CPMP/040/98 (10 March).
—— (1998c) 'CPMP opinion following an Article 10 referral – Amaryl (international non-proprietary name (INN) Glimepiride)', CPMP/1416/98 (3 August).

——— (1999a) 'Notice to marketing authorisation holders: pharmacovigilance guidelines', CPMP/PhVWP/108/99corr. (29 January).
——— (1999b) 'Scientific advice: role and responsibilities of the "Scientific Advice Review Group"', CPMP/180/99 (22 February).
——— (1999c) Press release on CPMP meeting held 22–23 June 1999, 25 June, CPMP/1817/99.
——— (1999d) 'CPMP joint pilot plan for the implementation of the electronic transmission of individual case safety reports between the EMEA, National Competent Authorities and the pharmaceutical industry', CPMP/PhVWP/2058/99 (29 July).
——— (1999e) 'Report on withdrawn centralised applications 1995–1998', EMEA/H/14994/99.
——— (1999f) World Wide Web URL http://www.eudra.org/emea.htm
——— (1999g) Fourth General Report on the Activities of the European Agency for the Evaluation of Medicinal Products, 1998. EMEA: London.
Epstein, S. (1996) Impure Science: AIDS, Activism, and the Politics of Knowledge. Berkeley: University of California Press.
——— (1997) 'Activism, drug regulation, and the politics of therapeutic evaluation in the AIDS era: a case study of ddC and the "surrogate markers" debate', Social Studies of Science, 27: 691–726.
Etzkowitz, H. and Webster, A. (1995) 'Science as intellectual property' in S. Jasanoff, G.E. Markle, J.C. Petersen and T. Pinch (eds) Handbook of Science and Technology Studies. Thousand Oaks: Sage, pp. 480–505.
European Commission (1965) Directive 65/65/EEC.
——— (1975a) Council Directive 75/318/EEC.
——— (1975b) Council Directive 75/319/EEC.
——— (1983) Directive 83/570/EEC.
——— (1985) Completing the Internal Market. White Paper from the Commission to the European Parliament, 6 March.
——— (1987) Directive 87/22/EEC.
——— (1989) Rules Governing Medicinal Products in the European Community Vol. 1, Preface. EC: Brussels.
——— (1993a) Directive 93/39/EEC.
——— (1993b) Council Regulation 2309/93/EEC.
——— (1994) Rules Governing Medicinal Products in the European Union Vol. 1. EC: Brussels.
——— (1995) Council Directive 540/95.
——— (1996a) Rules Governing Medicinal Products in the European Community Vol. IIA (Notice to Applicants). EC: Brussels.
——— (1996b) DGIII, 'Pharmaceuticals – mutual recognition procedure', press release, 21 March, Brussels.
——— (1997) 'Mutual recognition procedure (draft)', DGIII, 23 May.
Fiorino, D.J. (1990) 'Citizen participation and environmental risk: a survey of institutional mechanisms', Science, Technology and Human Values, 15: 226–43.
Fischer, F. (1990) Technocracy and the Politics of Expertise. London: Sage.
Frankenfield, P.J. (1992) 'Technological citizenship: a normative framework for risk studies', Science, Technology and Human Values, 17: 459–84.
Funtowicz, S.O. and Ravetz, J. (1993) 'Science for the post-normal age', Futures, 25: 740–57.
Gabe, J. and Bury, M. (1996) 'Halcion nights: a sociological account of a medical controversy', Sociology, 30: 447–69.
General Accounting Office (GAO) (1990) FDA Drug Review: Post-approval Risks 1976–85. Report to the Chairman, Subcommittee on Human Resources and Intergovernmental Relations, Committee on Government Operations, House of Representatives. GAO/PEMD–90–15.
Gieryn, T.F. (1983) 'Boundary-work and the demarcation of science from non-science: strains and interests in professional ideologies of scientists', American Sociological Review, 48: 781–95.
Gould, D. (1972) 'Sir Derrick Dunlop – noblesse oblige?' New Scientist (23 March): 626.

Grande, E. (1996) 'The state and interest groups in a framework of multi-level decision-making: the case of the European Union', *Journal of European Public Policy*, 3: 318–38.

Greenwood, J. and Ronit, K. (1991) 'Pharmaceutical regulation in Denmark and the UK', *European Journal of Political Research*, 19: 327–59.

Griffin, J.P. and Diggle, G.E. (1981) 'A survey of products licensed in the UK from 1971–81', *British Journal of Clinical Pharmacology*, 12: 453–63.

Griffin, J.P. and Long, J.R. (1981) 'New procedures affecting the conduct of clinical trials in the UK', *British Medical Journal*, 283: 477–9.

Haas, E. (1958) *The Uniting of Europe: Political, Social and Economic Forces, 1950–1957*. Stanford: Stanford University Press.

—— (1961) 'International integration: the European and the universal process', *International Organisation*, 15: 366–92.

Haas, P. (1992) 'Introduction: knowledge, power and international policy co-ordination', *International Organization*, 46 (special edition): 1–35.

HAI (Health Action International) (1992) *Secrecy Campaign Information Pack*. HAI: Amsterdam.

—— (1996) *Statement of the International Working Group on Transparency and Accountability in Drug Regulation*. Uppsala: Dag Hammarskjold Foundation.

—— (1997) 'Openness, the rule, secrecy the exception', press release, 30 October.

Hancher, L. (1989) 'Regulating for competition: government, law and the pharmaceutical industry in the UK and France', PhD thesis, University of Amsterdam.

—— (1996) 'Pharmaceutical policy and regulation: setting the pace in the European Community' in P. Davis (ed.) *Contested Ground: Public and Private Interests in the Regulation of Prescription Drugs*. New York: Oxford University Press.

Hancher, L. and Moran, M. (1989a) 'Introduction' in L. Hancher and M. Moran (eds) *Capitalism, Culture and Economic Regulation*. Oxford: Clarendon, pp. 1–10.

—— (1989b) 'Conclusion: organising regulatory space' in L. Hancher and M. Moran (eds) *Capitalism, Culture and Economic Regulation*. Oxford: Clarendon, pp. 271–300.

—— (eds) (1989c) *Capitalism, Culture and Economic Regulation*. Oxford: Clarendon.

Hancher, L. and Reute, M. (1984) 'Legal administrative culture as policy determinants: licensing and the drug industry'. Paper presented at ESRC Conference on Government Industry Relations in Major OECD Countries, Cambridge, 11 December.

Heads of Medicines Agency (1996) Statement, Meeting of Heads of Medicines Agencies of Member States, 23 February, the Netherlands.

Heritier, A. (1996) 'The accommodation of diversity in European policy-making and its outcomes: regulatory policy as patchwork', *Journal of European Public Policy*, 3: 149–67.

—— (1997) 'Policy-making by subterfuge: interest accommodation, innovation and substitute democratic legitimation in Europe', *Journal of European Public Policy*, 4: 171–89.

Hildebrandt, A.G. (1995a) 'Guest interview – the role of the German BfArM within the new EC regulatory framework (1),' *Regulatory Affairs Journal* (October): 813–17.

—— (1995b) 'Guest interview – the role of the German BfArM within the new EC regulatory framework (2)', *Regulatory Affairs Journal* (November): 909–13.

Hodgkin, C. (1996) 'Harmonising drug policy: making rules for tomorrow's market', *HAI-Lights*, 1: 2–3.

Holford, N.H.G. (1995) 'The target concentration approach to clinical drug development', *Clinical Pharmacokinetics*, 29: 287–91.

Holmes, P. (1999) 'Regulatory sovereignty in the EU and the WTO', *Euroscope*, 15: 2–3.

Hurley, R. (1983) 'The Medicines Act – is it working?' *Journal of the British Institute of Regulatory Affairs*, 2: 1–5.

Inman, W.H.W. (1986) *Monitoring for Drug Safety*. Lancaster: MTP Press.

International Federation of Pharmaceutical Industry Associations (IFPIA) (1998) 'Safety topics' in *ICH Topics and Guidelines* at http://www.ifpma.org/ich1.html

International Society of Drug Bulletins (ISDB) (1997) 'Transparency and openness: consultation on transparency and access to documentation at the EMEA', 11 April.

Irwin, A. (1995) *Citizen Science: A Study of People, Expertise and Sustainable Development*. London: Routledge.

Irwin, A., Rothstein, H., Yearley, S. and McCarthy, E. (1997) 'Regulatory science – towards a sociological framework', *Futures*, 29: 17–31.

Jasanoff, S. (1987) 'Contested boundaries in policy-relevant science', *Social Studies of Science*, 17: 195–230.

—— (1990) *The Fifth Branch: Science Advisers as Policymakers*. Cambridge, Massachusetts: Harvard University Press.

Jefferys, D. (1992) 'Simplifying drug licensing', *Scrip Magazine* (May): 12.

Jefferys, D. and Jones, K.H. (1995) 'EMEA and the new pharmaceutical procedures for Europe', *European Journal of Clinical Pharmacology*, 47: 471–6.

Jessop, B. (1990) *State Theory: Putting Capitalist States in Their Place*. Cambridge: Polity Press.

Jones, K. and Jefferys, D. (1994) 'EMEA and the new pharmaceutical procedures for Europe', *Health Trends*, 26 (1): 10–13.

Juillet, Y. (1994) 'The broader perspective' in Z. Bankowski and J.F. Dunne (eds) *Drug Surveillance: International Co-operation, Past, Present and Future*, (Proceedings of the XXVIIth CIOMS Conference, Geneva, Switzerland, 14–15 September 1994). CIOMS: Geneva.

Kelman, S. (1981) *Regulating Sweden, Regulating America: A Comparative Study of Occupational Safety and Health Policy*. Cambridge, Massachusetts: MIT Press.

Kendall, H.W. (1991) 'The failure of nuclear power' in M. Shubk (ed.) *Risk, Organisations and Society*. Boston: Kluwer, pp. 163–218.

Kerwin, K.W. and Travis, M.J. (1996) 'Side effects of pill scare', *Guardian*, 22 November.

Laird, F.N. (1993) 'Participatory analysis, democracy and technological decision making', *Science, Technology and Human Values*, 18: 341–61.

Lawson, D.H. (1984) 'Pharmacoepidemiology: a new discipline', *British Medical Journal*, 284: 940–41.

Lee, P. and Herzstein, J. (1986) 'International drug regulation', *Annual Review of Public Health*, 7: 217–35.

Lesser, F. (1977) 'Drug warnings', *New Scientist*, 78: 442.

Levidow, L., Carr, S., Wield, D. and von Schomberg, R. (1997) 'European biotechnology regulation: framing the risk assessment of a herbicide-tolerant crop', *Science, Technology and Human Values*, 22: 472–505.

Lewin, L. (1994) 'The rise and decline of corporatism: the case of Sweden', *European Journal of Political Research*, 26: 59–79.

Lexchin, J. (1990) 'Drug makers and drug regulators: too close for comfort', *Social Science and Medicine*, 31: 1257–63.

—— (1994) 'Who needs faster drug approval times in Canada: the public or the industry?' *International Journal of Health Services*, 24: 253–64.

Lexchin, J. and Kawachi, I. (1996) 'The self-regulation of pharmaceutical marketing initiatives for reform' in P. Davis (ed.) *Contested Ground: Public Purpose and Private Interest in the Regulation of Prescription Drugs*. New York/Oxford: Oxford University Press, pp. 221–35.

Liljestrand, A. (1979) 'Requirements in Sweden' in J.Z. Bowers and G.P. Velo (eds) *Drug Assessment Criteria and Methods*. Amsterdam: Elsevier, pp. 29–37.

Lindberg, L.N. (1963) *The Political Dynamics of European Economic Integration*. Stanford: Stanford University Press.

Lindroos, M. (1996) 'Nordic Council of Medicines (NLN)', *Regulatory Affairs Journal* (June): 464–6.

Litchfield, J.T. (1961) 'Forecasting drug effects in man from studies in laboratory animals', *Journal of the American Medical Association*, 8: 33–8.

Lumley, C.E. and Walker, S.R. (1985) 'A toxicology databank based on animal safety evaluation studies of pharmaceutical compounds', *Human Toxicology*, 4: 447–60.

Lumley, C.E., Parkinson, C. and Walker, S.R. (1993) 'The value of the dog in long-term toxicity studies: the CMR international toxicology database', *Adverse Drug Reaction Toxicology Review*, 12: 543–61.

MCA (Medicines Control Agency) (1991a) *Medicines Control Agency: Framework Document*. London: HMSO.

—— (1991b) *Commitment to Safety, Quality and Efficacy*. London: HMSO.

—— (1993a) *Towards Safe Drugs: A Guide to the Control of Safety, Quality and Efficacy of Human Medicines in the United Kingdom*. London: MCA.

—— (1993b) *MCA Annual Report and Accounts 1992/93*. London: HMSO.

—— (1995) *Annual report for 1994/95*. London: HMSO.

—— (1996) *MAIL 95* (May/June). London: HMSO.

—— (1997) *MCA Annual Report for 1996*. London: MCA.

McAuslane, N. (1996) 'International regulatory review times converge', *Centre for Medicines Research News*, 14: 1–2.

McDonell, G. (1997) 'Scientific and everyday knowledge: trust and the politics of environmental initiatives', *Social Studies of Science*, 27: 819–63.

McGowan, F. and Wallace, H. (1996) 'Towards a European regulatory state', *Journal of European Public Policy*, 3: 560–76.

Majone, G. (1994) 'The rise of the regulatory state in Europe', *West European Politics*, 17: 77–101.

—— (1996) *Regulating Europe*. London: Routledge.

Mann, R.D. (ed.) (1987) *Adverse Drug Reactions: The Scale and Nature of the Problem and the Way Forward*. Carnforth, England: Pathenon.

Medawar, C. (1984) *The Wrong Kind of Medicine?* London: Hodder and Stoughton.

—— (1992a) *Power and Dependence: Social Audit on the Safety of Medicines*. London: Social Audit.

—— (1992b) *Secrecy in Medicines*, HAI Secrecy Campaign Information Pack. HAI: Amsterdam.

—— (1996) 'Secrecy and medicines', *International Journal of Risk and Safety in Medicine*, 9: 133–41.

*Medicines Act* (1968). London: HMSO.

Merton, R.K. (1942) 'The normative structure of science' in N. Storer (ed.) *The Sociology of Science: Theoretical and Empirical Investigations*. Chicago: University of Chicago Press, pp. 267–78.

Middlemas, K. (1979) *Politics in Industrial Society: The Experience of the British System since 1911*. London: André Deutsch.

Millstone, E. (1986) *Food Additives*. Harmondsworth: Penguin.

Mintzes, B. and Hodgkin, C. (1996) 'The consumer movement: from single-issue campaigns to long-term reform' in P. Davis (ed.) *Contested Ground: Public Purpose and Private Interest in the Regulation of Prescription Drugs*. New York/Oxford: Oxford University Press, pp. 76–94.

Mitnick, B.M. (1980) *The Political Economy of Regulation*. New York: Columbia University Press.

Montanari, I.J. (1995) 'Harmonisation of social policies and social regulation in the European Community', *European Journal of Political Research*, 27: 21–45.

Moore, T.J. (1995) *Deadly Medicine: Why Tens of Thousands of Heart Patients Died in America's Worst Drug Disaster*. New York: Simon and Schuster.

Morgenstern, E. (1994) 'BGA restructure: update', *Regulatory Affairs Journal* (July): 582.

MPA (Medical Products Agency) (1996a) *The Medical Products Agency*, Uppsala: Lakemedelsverket.

—— (1996b) *MPA – A Professional Organisation*. Uppsala: Lakemedelsverket.

Mutual Recognition Facilitation Group (MRFG) (1999) Heads of Medical Agencies, World Wide Web URL: http://heads.medagencies.org/

National Consumer Council (NCC) (1993) *Balancing Acts: Conflicts of Interest in the Regulation of Medicines*. London: NCC.

—— (1994) *Secrecy and Medicines in Europe*. London: NCC.

Nelkin, D. (1984) *Science as Intellectual Property*. Washington DC: American Association for the Advancement of Science.

Offe, C. (1973) *Structural Problems of the Capitalist States*. Frankfurt: Suhrkamp.

Ollila, E. and Hemminki, E. (1996) 'Secrecy in drug regulation: licensing documentation on the Norplant contraceptive', *International Journal of Risk and Safety in Medicine*, 9: 161–72.

Owen, B. and Braeutigam, R. (1978) *The Regulation Game: Strategic Use of the Administrative Process*. Cambridge, Massachusetts: Ballinger Publishing Company.

Parkinson, C. (1992) 'Twelve month non-rodent studies debated at international forum', *CMR News*, 10, 1–3.

Peacock, A. (1984) *The Regulation Game*. Oxford: Basil Blackwell.

Pearce, N. (1996) 'Adverse reactions, social responses: a tale of two asthma mortality epidemics' in P. Davis (ed.) *Contested Ground: Public Purpose and Private Interest in the Regulation of Prescription Drugs*. New York/Oxford: Oxford University Press, pp. 57–75.

Peltzman, S. (1976) 'Toward a more general theory of regulation', *Journal of Economics and Law*, 19: 211–40.

Perhac, R.M. (1998) 'Comparative risk assessment: where does the public fit in?' *Science, Technology and Human Values*, 23: 221–41.

Personal communication (1996a) Electronic message from E. Koskinen, EMEA to G. Lewis, 14 May.

Personal communication (1996b) Letter from Dr D. Lyons, Irish National Medicines Board, to G. Lewis, 5 September.

Personal communication (1996c) Letter from G. Ekbom, Senior Legal Officer, MPA, to G. Lewis, 27 June.

Rawlins, M.D. (1988) 'Spontaneous reporting of adverse drug reactions', *British Journal of Clinical Pharmacology*, 16: 1–11.

—— (1993) 'Pharmacovigilance: paradise lost, regained or postponed?' *Journal of Clinical Pharmacology*, 35: 599–602.

—— (1994) 'The broader perspective' in Z. Bankowski and J.F. Dunne (eds) *Drug Surveillance: International Cooperation, Past, Present and Future* (Proceedings of the XXVIIth CIOMS Conference, Geneva, Switzerland, 14–15 September). Geneva: CIOMS, pp. 34–7.

—— (1996) 'A heavy dose: doctors and new drugs under surveillance', *Guardian*, 25 November.

Rawlins, M. and Jefferys, D. (1993) 'UK licensing trends', *British Journal of Clinical Pharmacology*, 35: 599–602.

Rawlins, M.D., Fracchia, G.N. and Rodriguez-Farre, E. (1992) 'EURO-ADR: pharmacovigilance and research: a European perspective', *Pharmacoepidemiology and Drug Safety*, 1: 261–8.

Richards, E. (1991) *Vitamin C and Cancer: Medicine or Politics?* London: Macmillan.

Robertson, K. (1982) *Public Secrets*. London: Macmillan.

Salsburg, D. (1983) 'The lifetime feeding study in mice and rats – an examination of its validity as a bioassay for human carcinogens', *Fundamental and Applied Toxicology*, 3: 63–8.

Salter, L. (1988) *Mandated Science: Science and Scientists in the Making of Standards*. Dordrecht: Kluwer.

Schmitter, P. C. (1974) 'Still the century of corporatism?' *Review of Politics*, 36: 85–131.

Schmitt-Rau, K. (1988) 'The drug regulatory system in the FRG', *Journal of Clinical Pharmacology*, 28: 1064–70.

Schwartzmann, D. (1976) *Innovation in the Pharmaceutical Industry*. Baltimore: Johns Hopkins University.

Siehr, K.G. (1986) 'Drug reactions and the law in the European Community' in W.H.W. Inman (ed.) *Monitoring for Drug Safety*. Lancaster, England; MTP Press.

Skea, J. and Christensen, S. (1991) *Acid Politics: Environmental and Energy Policies in Britain and Germany*. London: Belhaven Press.

Smart, R.D. (1981) 'Foreword' in *ABPI Annual Report for 1980–81*. London: ABPI, p. 3.

Stigler, G.J. (1971) 'The theory of economic regulation', *Bell Journal of Economics and Management Science*, 2: 3–21.

Stone-Sweet, A. and Sandholtz, W. (1997) 'European integration and supranational governance', *Journal of European Public Policy*, 4: 1–23.

Tuffs, A. (1993) 'Ideas for BGA reform', *Lancet*, 342 (11 December): 1479.

US Congress (1970) 'The British drug safety system', *Twenty-second Report Committee on Government Operations*. Washington DC: US GPO.

Vaughan, D. (1989) 'Regulating risk: implications of the Challenger accident', *Law and Policy*, 11: 330–49.

Vogel, D. (1995) *Trading Up: Consumer and Environmental Regulation in a Global Economy*. Cambridge, Massachusetts: Harvard University Press.

—— (1998) 'The globalization of pharmaceutical regulation', *Governance*, 11: 1–22.

Wade, O.L. (1983) 'Achievements, problems and limitations of regulatory bodies' in B. Farrell (ed.) *Medicines Review Worldwide – A Patient Benefit or a Regulatory Burden? Proceedings of the Fifth Annual Symposium of the British Institute of Regulatory Affairs*. London: British Institute of Regulatory Affairs, pp. 2–9.

Walker, J.W. (1993) *Dirty Medicine: Science, Big Business and the Assault on Natural Health Care*. London: Slingshot Publications.

Walker, S.R. and Lumley, C.E. (1987) 'Reporting and under-reporting' in R.D. Mann (ed.) *Adverse Drug Reactions: The Scale and Nature of the Problem and the Way Forward*. Carnforth, England: Pathenon.

Weinberg, A.M. (1972) 'Science and trans-science', *Minerva*, 10: 209–22.

Whitley, R. (1992) *European Business Systems: Firms and Markets in their National Contexts*. London: Sage.

Wilks, S. (1996) 'Regulatory compliance and capitalist diversity in Europe', *Journal of European Public Policy*, 3: 536–59.

Williams, G. and Popay, J. (1994) 'Lay knowledge and the privilege of experience' in J. Gabe, D. Kelleher and G. Williams (eds) *Challenging Medicine*. London: Routledge.

Wilson, G.M. (1962) 'Assessing new drugs', *New Scientist* (26 July): 196.

Wilson, J.Q. (ed.) (1980) *The Politics of Regulation*. New York: Basic Books.

Wood, S. (1996) Presentation to Third Annual Conference of Regulatory Authorities, February, London.

World Health Organisation (WHO) (1969) 'Principles for the testing and evaluation of drugs for carcinogenicity', *Technical Report Series* No. 426. WHO: Geneva.

—— (1974) 'Assessment of the carcinogenicity and mutagenicity of chemicals', *Technical Report Series* No. 546. WHO: Geneva.

World Health Organisation Working Group on Clinical Pharmacology in Europe (1988) 'Clinical pharmacology in Europe – an indispensable part of the health service', *European Journal of Clinical Pharmacology*, 33: 535–9.

Wright Mills, C. (1959) *The Power Elite*. New York: Oxford University Press.

Wyatt-Walter, A. (1995) 'Globalization, corporate identity and European technology policy', *Journal of European Public Policy*, 2: 427–46.

Wynne, B. (1980) 'Technology, risk and participation: on the social treatment of uncertainty' in J. Conrad (ed.) *Society, Technology and Risk Assessment*. London: Academic Press.

—— (1995) 'Public understanding of science' in S. Jasanoff, G.E. Markle, J.C. Petersen and T. Pinch (eds) *Handbook of Science and Technology Studies*. Thousand Oaks: Sage, pp. 361–88.

Zahn, M. (1994) 'BGA disbanded: Healthcare Institutions Reform Act published', *Regulatory Affairs Journal* (August): 669–70.

—— (1995) 'BfArM letter to VFA', *Regulatory Affairs Journal* (December): 1056.

Zbinden, G. (1987) 'Predictive values of animal studies in toxicology', Centre for Medicines Research lecture, Carshalton, England.

# Index